Diabetic Retinopathy:
Introduction to
Novel Treatment Strategies

Dr. Deepa Pathak

M.Pharm, Ph.D

Women Scientist-A (DST, New Delhi)
J.S.S. College of Pharmacy,
Udhagamandalm, T.N.-643001

and

Dr. K. Gowthamarajan

M.Pharm, Ph.D

Head in Pharmaceutics,
J.S.S. College of Pharmacy,
Udhagamandalm, India.

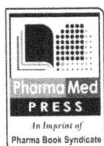

PharmaMed Press

An imprint of Pharma Book Syndicate

A Unit of BSP Books Pvt. Ltd.

4-4-309/316, Giriraj Lane,

Sultan Bazar, Hyderabad - 500 095.

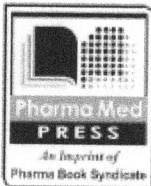

Published by

PharmaMed Press

An imprint of Pharma Book Syndicate

A Unit of BSP Books Pvt. Ltd.

4-4-309/316, Giriraj Lane, Sultan Bazar, Hyderabad - 500 095.

Phone: 040-23445605, 23445688; Fax: 91+40-23445611

E-mail: info@pharmamedpress.com

ISBN: 978-93-85433-64-1 (HB)

PREFACE

Diabetic retinopathy (DR) still represents one of the leading causes of vision loss worldwide. Since this condition affects the posterior segment of the eye, topical application of ophthalmic medicines is of limited benefit, considering that they seldom reach therapeutic levels in the affected tissues. Systemic medications can be insufficient due to the eye's immunoprivileged condition and existence of both inner and outer blood-retinal barriers, which place limitations on the potential role of this route of administration for retinal diseases.

In this setting, intraocular therapies have emerged as novel and vital tools in the ophthalmologist's armamentarium against DR, allowing for maximization of drug efficacy and limited risk of systemic side effects. Intravitreal injections have been widely used for treating DR particularly in the 21 (st) centuries.

Other agents targeting molecules, such as anti-vascular endothelial growth factor, have also demonstrated a potential therapeutic role for treatment.

Recent advances in ocular drug delivery methods have led to the development of intraocular implants, which help to provide prolonged treatment with controlled drug release. Moreover, they may add some potential advantages over traditional intraocular injections by delivering certain rates of drug directly to the site of action, amplifying the drug's half-life, contributing in the minimization of peak plasma levels of the drug, and avoiding the side effects associated with repeated intravitreal injections.

The Diabetic Retinopathy: Introduction to Novel Treatment Strategy is the most recent book in the area of novel delivery systems for the treatment of diabetic retinopathy. For many years, interest has been expressed in optimizing drug therapy through intravitreal injection delivery system design. In this modern era there has been move away from costly and nonpatient compliance treatment through development of more advance drug delivery system and manufacturing techniques and rely on novel means for controlling the release of drug form the delivery system, cost effective and patient compliance. This is an exciting and growing area of pharmaceutical research and till date very less information is available on novel delivery system for the treatment of diabetic retinopathy. Therefore, we decided to edit a book comprised of chapters that collectively address this void and provide an insight into various approaches for the treatment of diabetic retinopathy.

The book is divided into different chapters, each of which addresses introduction to novel drug delivery systems with suitable scientific examples and carefully edited for academia and industry need based to bring a new challenge novel and cost effective /patient friendly delivery systems.

The book **Diabetic Retinopathy: Introduction to Novel Treatment Strategies** will certainly stands as the landmark on Diabetic Retinopathy.

Authors -

ACKNOWLEDGEMENT

We would like to thank Department of Science and Technology, New Delhi, India for providing financial assistance for carrying out project about novel approaches for the treatment of diabetic retinopathy. We also thank J.S.S. College of Pharmacy, Udhagamandalm, India for providing facilities to carry out this research.

CONTENTS

CHAPTER 5

VARIOUS OCULAR DRUG DELIVERY SYSTEMS

CHAPTER 6

NOVEL STRATEGIES FOR THE TREATMENT OF DIABETIC RETINOPATHY

CHAPTER 7

FUTURE PROSPECTIVE

CHAPTER 1

INTRODUCTION AND SYMPTOMS

Introduction of Diabetic Retinopathy

Diabetic retinopathy (DR) is a potentially blinding complication of diabetes. It is defined as presence of one or more definite microaneurism or any other more severe lesion formed in any stage of retinopathy. Retinopathy frequently appears after 5 years of untreated diabetes and 50% of patients have some evidence of it in less than 10 years. At first, there is no changes in your vision and could get worse over the years and threaten your vision. With timely treatment, 90% of those with advanced diabetic retinopathy can be saved from going blind. Everyone with diabetes should have an eye examination through dilated pupils at least once a year. DR occurs when diabetes damages the tiny blood vessels inside the retina, the light sensitive tissue at the back of the eye. At this point, most people do not notice any changes in their vision. Some people develop a condition called macular oedema. It occurs when the damaged blood vessels leak fluid and lipids on to the macula, the part of the retina. The fluid makes the macula swells and blurring of vision takes place. As the disease progress it enters an advanced proliferative stage. Retinopathy before the development of retinal neovascularization is termed nonproliferative diabetic retinopathy (NPDR). Once proliferation of new retinal vessel occurs, it is referred to as proliferative diabetic retinopathy (PDR)[1].

In 1967, in his magnum opus *"The system of Ophtalmology, Sir Stewart Duke-Elder had written,"....diabetic retinopathy is one of the major tragedies of ophthalmology in our present generation; always common and rapidly becoming still more common; affecting the young as well as the aged, predictable but not preventable."*

Stages and Symptoms of Diabetic Retinopathy

There are four stages of diabetic retinopathy these are;

1. **Mild Nonproliferative Retinopathy (NPDR):** It is earliest stage of retinopathy and at this stage balloon like swelling takes place in the small area of retinal blood vessels.

2. **Moderate Nonproliferative Retinopathy:** It is the second stage and at this stage some blood vessels nourish the retina get blocked.

3. **Severe Nonproliferative Retinopathy:** At this third stage more blood vessels get blocked.

4. **Proliferative Retinopathy (PDR):** At this advanced stage due to retinal ischemia, hypoxic condition occur and a signal sent by the retina for nourishment, cause the growth of new blood vessels, this condition is called neovascularization. These newly formed blood vessels have fragile and thin walled, leak the blood on the surface of eye and blindness takes place. Retinal neovascularization, a hallmark of proliferative diabetic retinopathy (PDR), is a major risk factor for severe vision loss in patients[2]. Depending on the degree and severity of retinal new vessels, presence of vitreous or pre-retinal hemorrhage and retinal detachment, PDR can be categorized as nonproliferative diabetic retinopathy (Pericyte loss, basement membrane thickening, vascular leakage, alteration in blood flow, tissue hypoxia), preproliferative diabetic retinopathy (Hypoxia, oedema, microaneurysms, soft exudates, venous beading) and proliferative diabetic retinopathy (Angiogenesis, fibrovascular ridge, breakdown of inner blood-retinal barrier, retinal detachment, blindness). The various stages and their symptoms were shown in Table 1.1 and Figure 1.1.

Table 1.1 Clinical stages and symptoms of diabetic retinopathy.

S. No.	Disease Level	Lesions Finding
1	No apparent retinopathy	No abnormalities.
2	Mild NPDR	Microaneurysm only.
3	Moderate NPDR	More than just microaneurism but less than severe NPDR
4	Severe NPDR	No sign of PDR, with any of the following: Intra retinal hemorrhages, venous beading and intra retinal microvascular anomalies.
5	Low-risk PDR	New vessels elsewhere>0.5 disc area in 1 or more quadrants.

Contd...

S. No.	Disease Level	Lesions Finding
6	Moderate-risk PDR	New vessels elsewhere$\geq$0.5 disc area in 1 or more quadrants or new vessels on disc <0.25-0.33 disc area either new vessels on disc.
7	High-risk PDR	<0.25-0.33 disc area or new vessels elsewhere <0.5 disc area and vitreous hemorrhage. New vessels on disc $\geq$0.25-0.33 disc area (with or without vitreous hemorrhage). New vessels elsewhere > 1 disc area (with or without vitreous hemorrhage).
8	Advanced PDR	Traction, retinal detachment, rubeosisiridis, fundus partially obscured.

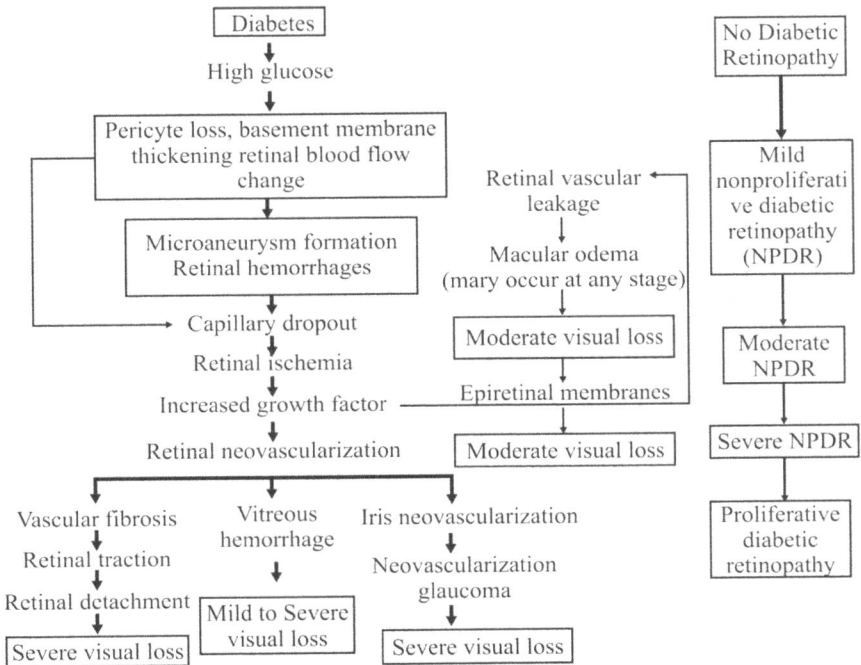

Fig. 1.1 Various stages and their symptoms of diabetic retinopathy.

In DR elevated level of $HbA_{1\alpha}$ and reduced level of 2, 3-diphosphoglycerate decreased the release of O_2 from Hb which causes retinal hypoxia and ischemia. In early stage retinal ischemia is reversible and becomes irreversible if blood-retinal barrier breaks and tight endothelial junctions open up. The break down of blood retinal barrier is related to duration and severity of diabetes mellitus. Initially, in uncontrolled diabetes mellitus, there is compensatory increase in retinal blood volume and segmental blood flow along with auto regulatory dilation of retinal blood vessels. With development of diabetic retinopathy there is regional hyper perfusion of retina due to removal of floating matter where RBCs shunted through some capillaries and plasma alone. Eventually, severity of retinal hypoxia increases microaneurism, cotton-wool spot, new vessel formation (proliferative retinopathy), intra retinal oedema and hemorrhage. Thus, retinal manifestations of diabetes are- Microaneurysms (MA), Haemorrhages (H), Soft exudates (SE), Hard exudates (HE), Venous beading (VB), Intra retinal microvascular anomalies (IRMA), Neovascularisation elsewhere (NVE), Neovascularisation of the optic disc (NVD), Clinically significant macular oedema (CSME)[3].

Epidemiology

The biggest risk factor for diabetes is diabetes itself. The Indian figures for the prevalence of diabetic retinopathy vary from 4 to 28%. The WHO multinational study of vascular disease in diabetes estimated the prevalence of diabetic retinopathy in males and females as 6.25% and 4.5% respectively. In population study at a South Indian urban setting retinopathy was found in 87.55% of diabetes with duration more than 15 years compared to 18.9% in those with duration of disease less than 15 years. The incidence of the severity of diabetic retinopathy as seen in the South Indian study among recently detected diabetes revealed non-proliferative diabetic retinopathy at 30.8% including 6.4% with maculopathy and proliferative diabetic retinopathy at 3.4%. In a population based assessment of diabetes and diabetic retinopathy, the age-sex adjusted prevalence of diabetes among people aged 50 years and over was 5.1% and of diabetic retinopahy among diabetes was 26.8% with non-proliferative retinopathy being the most common form (94.1%). Puberty and pregnancy can accelerate retinopathy progression. The onset of vision-threatening retinopathy is rare in children before puberty regardless of the duration of diabetes. However, if diabetes is diagnosed between the ages of 10 and 30 years, significant retinopathy may arise within 6 years of the disease. Proliferative retinopathy is present in 25% of the patients with type 1 and the duration of 15 years but in 25% of the type 2 diseases at duration of 25 years. However, in type 2 diseases with less than five years proliferative retinopathy develops in 2% only. The prevalence of macular oedema is approximately 18 to 19% in patients either with type 1 disease or type 2[4].

Diabetes is one of the most serious challenges to health care world-wide. According to recent projections it will affect 239 million people by 2010 doubling in prevalence since 1994. Diabetes will affect 28 million in Western Europe, 18.9 million in North America, 138.2 million in Asia and 1.3 million in Australia. The prevalence of blindness due to DR in Western Communities is estimated as between 1.6-1.9/ 100,000 about 8% of UK registrations are due to diabetes. Diabetes mellitus is the most common cause of blindness amongst individuals of working-age (20-65 years).

References

1. Aiello LP, Gardner TW, King GL, Blankenship G, Cavallerano JD, Ferris FL, Klein R, Diabetic Retinopathy (Technical review), Dia Care, 1998, 1, 48-61.

2. Derubertis FR and Craven PA, Activation of protein kinase C in glomerular cells in diabetes: Mechanism and potential link to the pathogenesis of diabetic glomerulopathy, Diabetes, 1994, 43, 1-8.

3. Baynes J.W, Role of oxidative stress in development of complications in diabetes, Diabetes, 1991, 40, 405-412.

4. Sachdev Y and Gupta DN, Clinical endocrinology and diabetes mellitus: A comprehensive text, volume 2, Jaypee brothers medical publishers (P) ltd., pp. 990-999.

CHAPTER 2

PATHOGENESIS AND
INVESTIGATIONS

Aetiopathogenesis

The key that opens all the mechanisms for development of diabetic retinopathy (DR) is ischemia. DR is characterized by the formation of primitive, leaky and disorganized vascular networks, which grow into the vitreous and reflect the unique aspects of vascular endothelial growth factor (VEGF) function which in turn is activated by the active protein kinase C (PKC) receptor. In hyperglycemic patients there is an increase in diacylglycerol generation (DAG), advance glycosylation end product (AGE) and free radical generation which activate PKC receptor by DAG-PKC pathway. The expression level of VEGF gets influenced by binding with hypoxia inducible factor (HIF-1α). In diabetic retinopathy oxygen supply to the part of retina is decreased which blocks the blood vessels due to this hypoxic and ischemic condition takes place and to compensate from this there is a formation of new blood vessels in presence of VEGF and HIF-1α expression, this condition is called neovascularization. These newly formed blood vessels are leaky, fragile and having thin wall which leak the blood on the surface of eye and blindness takes place[1-4].

DR progresses through various stages, the two main stages of visual loss/impairment in patients with diabetic retinopathy are: proliferative diabetic retinopathy (PDR) and diabetic macularoedema (DME). Retinal neovascularization, a hallmark of proliferative diabetic retinopathy (PDR), is a major risk factor for severe vision loss in patients. Depending on the degree and severity of formed new vessels, presence of vitreous or pre-retinal hemorrhage and retinal detachment, PDR **(Figure 2.1)** can be categorized as nonproliferative diabetic retinopathy (Pericyte loss, basement membrane thickening, vascular leakage, alteration in blood flow, tissue hypoxia), preproliferative diabetic retinopathy (Hypoxia, oedema, microaneurysms, soft exudates, venous beading) and proliferative diabetic retinopathy (angiogenesis, fibrovascular ridge, breakdown of inner blood-retinal barrier, retinal detachment, blindness). Diabetic macular edema (DME) is the most common cause of moderate visual loss which may be associated with any of the stages of retinopathy[5]. DME is defined as retinal thickening or presence of hard exudates within one disc diameter of the centre of the macula.

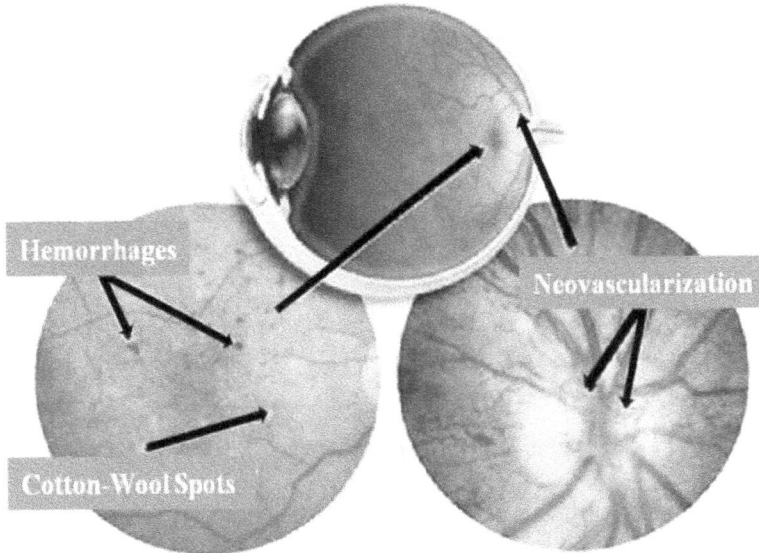

Fig. 2.1 The symptom from Preproliferative to Proliferative diabetic retinopathy.

The DAG-PKC pathway contributes to vascular function in many ways, such as regulation of endothelial permeability, vaso-constriction, extracellular matrix synthesis/turnover, cell growth, angiogenesis, cytokine activation and leucocyte adhesion[6-7]. The pathophysiology of DR was shown in **Figure 2.2.**

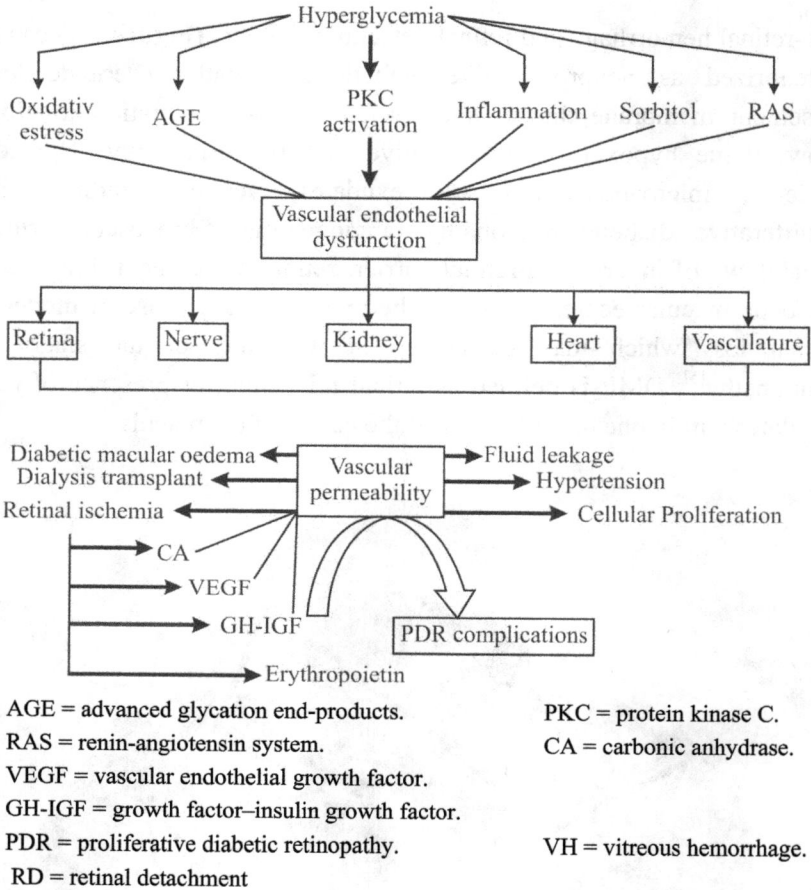

AGE = advanced glycation end-products.   PKC = protein kinase C.
RAS = renin-angiotensin system.   CA = carbonic anhydrase.
VEGF = vascular endothelial growth factor.
GH-IGF = growth factor–insulin growth factor.
PDR = proliferative diabetic retinopathy.   VH = vitreous hemorrhage.
 RD = retinal detachment

Fig. 2.2 Pathophysiology of diabetic retinopathy.

Pathogenesis of Diabetic Retinopathy and Characteristic Fundus Lesions

The clinical classification and types of lesions detected on fundoscopy are as follows[8]:

1. Non-proliferative Diabetic Retinopathy (NPDR)

(i) Mild non-proliferative diabetic retinopathy

- Microaneurysms
- Dot and blot haemorrhages
- Hard (intra-retinal) exudates

(ii) Moderate-to-severe non-proliferative diabetic retinopathy
- Cotton-wool spots
- Venous beading and loops
- Intraretinal microvascular abnormalities (IRMA)

2. Diabetic Retinopathy
- Neovascularization of the retina, optic disc or iris
- Fibrous tissue adherent to vitreous face of retina
- Retinal detachment
- Vitreous haemorrhage
- Pre retinal haemorrhage

3. Maculopathy
- Clinically significant macular oedema (CSME)
- Ischaemic Maculopathy

Microaneurysms (MA): These are small pinhead like, red looking lesions that are usually found in the macular area and around the disc. They are seen ophthalmoscopically as small dots usually varying from 10 to 15 micron in size. But they are clearly delineated after an intravascular injection of fluorescein in an area, which may have appeared as normal on ophthalmoscopy. In numbers, these microaneurysms vary from a few to an astonishing quantity scattered over the retina. They usually arise from the venous side of the capillary network, as localized distensions of the one side of the vessel wall, generally forming saccular diverticula full of blood; on the other hand, they may arise from the capillary loops, formed perhaps by endothelial proliferation and migration **(Figure 2.3).**

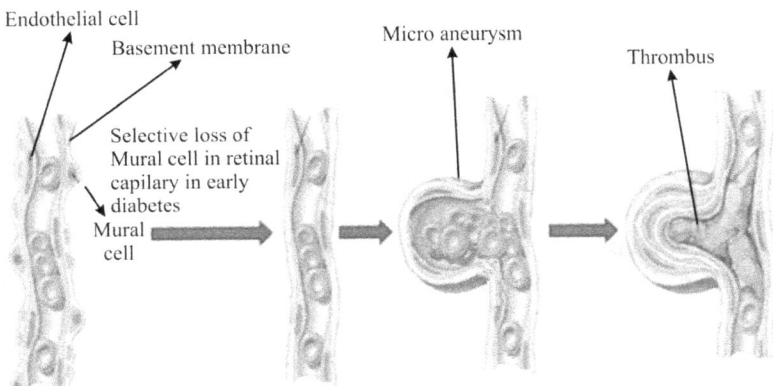

Out pouching which may be thin or may show endothelial proliferation or basement membrane thickening develop in capillary wall. Thrombosis may occur.

Fig. 2.3 Formation of Microaneurysm.

Haemorrhages (H): Haemorrhages in DR are usually intraretinal arising from deeper capillaries located within the compact inner nuclear and outer plexiform layers of the retina and thus assuming the typical dot and blot appearance. Haemorrhages occurring in the inner retina assume a flame shape due to the thicking of the blood between the nerve-fibre layers of the retina. Through they may be seen with many systemic and other retinal disorders, they are often associated with systemic hypertension and a plethora of these in a case of DR should lead to a suspicion of uncontrolled hypertension **(Figure 2.4)**.

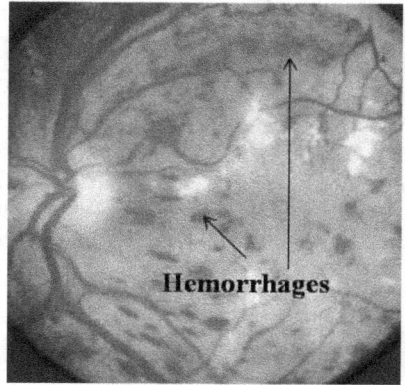

Fig. 2.4 Formation of Hemorrhages.

Soft Exudates (SE): Also known as cotton-wool spot, they are seen on ophthalmoscopy as discrete fluffy white like opacification in the inner retina. They represent swelling and disruption of axoplasmic flow within nerve-fiber layer and thus are signs of focal ischemia in the retina. However, they are less helpful in predicting progression to proliferative phase **(Figure 2.5)**.

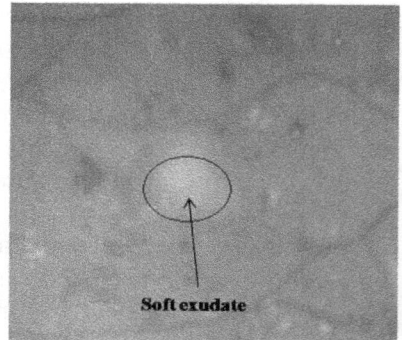

Fig. 2.5 Formation of Soft exudates.

Hard Exudates (HE): They have a waxy yellow appearance with sharply defined borders (as compared to the fluffy bordered SE) and represent the residue of oedema that has leaked from abnormal retinal vessels. HE tend to accumulate in the outer plexiform layer (hence deeper to SE), where the tissue is most lax. They usually assume a ring like or circinate conformation around the site of leakage, such as from a retinal microaneuryms or a diseased capillary leakage **(Figure 2.6)**.

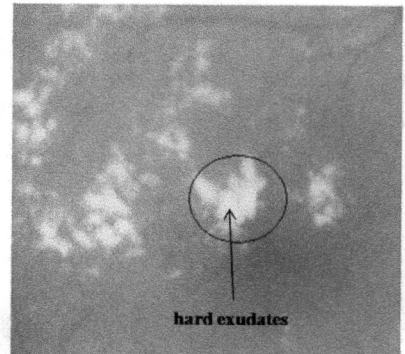

Fig. 2.6 Formation of Soft exudates.

Venous beading (VB): This is the term given to the beaded appearance of the veins that are dilated segments of retinal veins. The veins may also undergo tortuosity and reduplication.

Intraretinal Microvascular Abnormalities (IRMA): One of the most serious consequences of DR is the obliteration of retinal capillaries. When patches of cellular capillaries, seen early in the course of the disease, become confluent, the terminal arterioles that supply these capillaries often become occluded. Adjacent to these areas of non-perfused retina, clusters of MA and tortuous, hypercellular vessels often develop. It is difficult to determine whether these vessels are dilated pre-existing vessels or neovascularization in the retina. These vessels have been referred to as intraretinal microvascular abnormalities clinically to include both possibilities.

Neovascularisation: These are the new vessel proliferations seen in the retina. Their extent, location from the optic disc and their position within the retinal layers or on the surface of the retina represent the extent of ischemia **(Figure 2.7).**

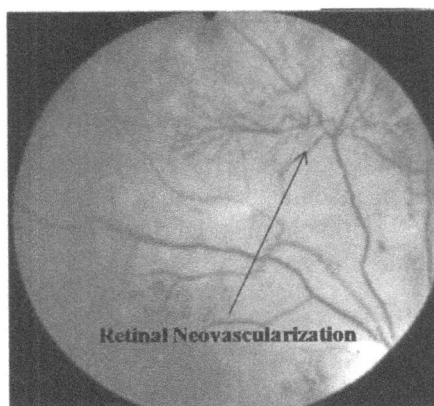

Fig. 2.7 Retinal neovascularization.

Neovascularization of the Optic Disc (NVD): The development of new vessels on the optic disc or up to 01 disc diopters of the optic disc is termed as neovascularization of the optic disc. The extent of the NVD represents the extent of retinal ischemia of at least five disc diopters of retinal area and its presence is of critical importance in a case of DR.

Diabetic Macular Oedema and Clinically Significant Macular Oedema: Retinal oedema threatening or involving the macula is an important visual consequence of abnormal retinal vascular permeability in DR because of the breakdown of the blood-retinal barrier. This is best delineated by fluorescein angiogram. Diabetic macular oedema may manifest as focal or diffuse retinal thickening with or without exudates. However, simple leakage on the angiogram may not always be associated with retinal thickening in the macular area. Although an overlap of categories often occurs two general categories of macular oedema, focal and diffuse.

Focal Macula Oedema: Areas of focal fluorescein leakage from specific capillary lesions characterize focal macular oedema. It may be associated with rings of hard exudates derived from plasma lipoproteins that appear to emanate from microaneurism. Resorption of fluid components results in precipitation of lipid residues, usually in the outer and inner plexiform layers but occasionally beneath the sensory retina itself (these are the hard exudates).

Diffuse Macular Oedema: Diffuse macular oedema is characterized by widespread retinal capillary abnormalities associated with diffuse leakage from extensive breakdown of blood-retinal-barrier and often with cystoids macular oedema. The diagnosis of macular oedema is best made by slit lamp biomicroscopy of the posterior pole using a noncontact 78D/90D or a Goldman contact lens. Important observations include-location of retinal oedema relative to the fovea, presence and location of exudates and presence of cystoids macular oedema.

However, the early Treatment Diabetic retinopathy Study (ETDRS) has thrown a pattern of macular oedema, which has been defined by the study as clinically significant macular oedema (CSME). Its common forms of presentation are as follows-

(a) Retinal oedema located at or within 500 μm of the centre of the macula.

(b) HE at or within 500 μm of the centre if associated with thickening of the adjacent retina.

(c) A zone of retinal thickening larger than 01 disc area if located within the 01 disc diameter of the center of the macula **(Figure 2.8).**

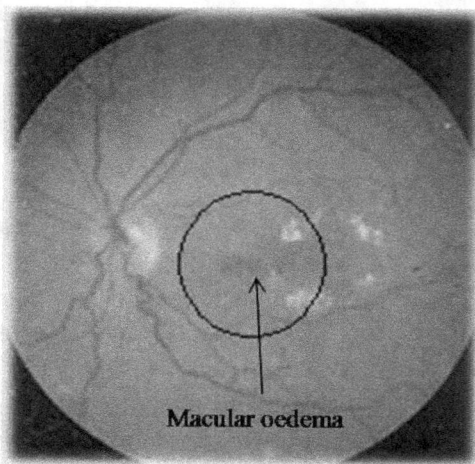

Macular oedema

Fig. 2.8 Diabetic Macular Oedema.

Causes of Diabetic Retinopathy[9-10]

1. **Glycosylated Proteins and Free Radicals:** One cause of many diabetic complications, including retinopathy, is the formation of glycosylated proteins and the resulting production of free radicals. Over time, if blood sugar is high, glucose can attach to protein such as hemoglobin. When this happens, the protein is glycosylated. Haemoglobin is just one of the proteins that can become generate free radicals, which cause oxidative stress, resulting in tissue damage. The body manufactures substances called antioxidants to neutralize free radicals. In the presence of too many free radicals, these natural neutralizers can become depleted e.g. glutathione, deficiency in retinas of diabetic and more malondialdehyde in oxidative stress. A subgroup of glycosylated proteins called advanced glycosylated end product (AGE) cause further damage by free radicals and also by combining with fats. They deposits in blood vessels, tissues, wreaking all sorts of havoc. AGE appears to contribute to the growth of new blood vessels in proliferative retinopathy. The activation of the DAG-PKC pathway is associated with many vascular abnormalities in the retina, renal and cardiovascular tissues in diabetic and insulin resistant states shown in **Figure 2.9**. The DAG-PKC pathway contributes to vascular function in many ways, such as the regulation of endothelial permeability, vasoconstriction, extracellular matrix (ECM) synthesis/turnover, cell growth, angiogenesis, cytokine activation and leucocyte adhesion.

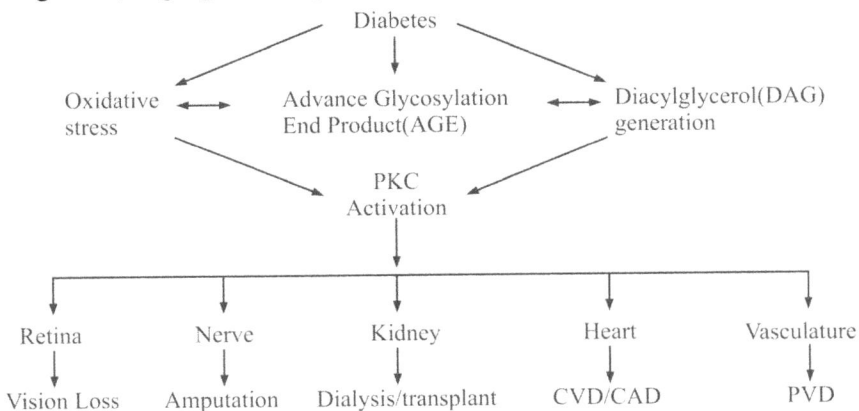

Fig. 2.9 Different abnormalities due to activation of DAG-PKC pathway.

2. **Lack of Oxygen to the Retina:** In diabetic retinopathy, oxygen supply to parts of the retina is decreased. This is primarily caused by blocked blood vessels. Furthermore, the red blood cells of people with

diabetes may be less flexible, particularly among those who have trouble keeping their blood sugar under control. The red blood cells need to change shape to fit through the tiny capillaries in the retina. If they can't do this, they may get stuck inside the narrowed vessels and created blockages, further reducing oxygen supply to certain areas of the retina. To compensate for the decreased oxygen, new vessels form, leading to the condition called proliferative retinopathy.

3. **Sorbitol Accumulation:** Researchers disagree as to weather accumulation of sorbitol, a glucose by product, is a cause of retinopathy. Substances called aldose reductase inhibitors, which prevent accumulation of Sorbitol, have been found to prevent retinopathy in studies of animals, but not in humans.

4. **Elevated Homocysteine Levels:** Homocysteine may also contribute to retinopathy, although the evidence is conflicting. The patients with retinopathy had abnormally high homocysteine levels, while those without retinopathy did not. It is believed that homocysteine can damage blood vessels, and this may be another mechanism leading to retinopathy. However, no correlation between retinopathy and high homocysteine levels except in the patients who also had kidney damage was reported.

Investigations

Diabetic retinopathy is detected during an eye examination by-

1. **Best Corrected Visual Acuity:** Quantitates level of high-contrast high frequency visual function. Decline can indicate onset of visually significant macular oedema, vitreous haemorrhage, cataract, macular traction detachment, etc.

2. **Ocular Alignment and Motility:** Evaluates function of oculomotor cranial nerves. Abnormalities can indicate ocular nerve abnormalities associated with diabetic nerve damage to cranial nerves III, IV, VI.

3. **Pupil Reactivity and Function:** Evaluates pupil-motor pathway and structural integrity of the iris. Abnormalities can indicate neuropathy, iris neovascularization, or afferent papillary defect.

4. **Visual Fields:** Evaluates possible defects in peripheral vision. Confrontational fields provide a qualitative assessment, and perimetry provides a quantitative assessment. Abnormalities can indicate vitreous/preretinal haemorrhage, retinal detachment and vascular occlusion.

5. **Intraocular Pressure:** For measurement of intraocular pressure application of tonometry is preferred, a standard test that determines the fluid pressure inside the eye. Abnormalities can indicate possible neovascular or open-angle glaucoma.

6. **Slit lamp Examination:**

    (i) Cornea: Assessment of ocular surface. Abnormalities can indicate epithelial abnormalities, defects, or infection.

    (ii) Iris: Assess iris and when indicated gonioscopy for possible angle-closure or angle neovascularization. Abnormalities can indicate neovascular glaucoma.

    (iii) Lens: Assess lens nucleus, cortex and posterior capsule. Abnormalities can indicate cataract.

    (iv) Vitreous: Assess clarity and character of vitreous gel. Abnormalities can indicate vitreous haemorrhage (red cells), retinal tear or detachment (pigment cells), or possible vitreoretinal traction.

7. **Dilated Funds Examination, Slit Lamp Biomicroscopy and Binocular Indirect Ophthalmoscopy:** This is an examination assess, presence, location and extent of retinovitreal disease in which the eye care professional; i) looks through a device with a special magnifying lens that provides a narrow view of the retina, or ii) wearing a headset with a bright light, looks through a special magnifying glass and gains a wide view of the retina.

8. **Fluorescein Angiography:** In this test, a special dye is injected into the arm. Pictures are then taken as the dye passes through the blood vessels in the retina. This test allows your doctor to find the leaking blood vessels. The benefits of this are-

    - *Guiding treatment of CSME:* Identification of treatable lesions and methods of photocoagulation.

    - *Determining extent of macular non-perfusion:* Extent and location may alter visual and treatment prognosis.

    - *Evaluating unexplained visual loss:* additional information.

    - *Searching for subtle neovascularization:* Rarely helpful as clinical examination is highly sensitive and HRC should usually be clinically identifiable.

    - *Diagnosis of NPDR:* In the absence of other indications.

- *Diagnosis of PDR before panretinal photocoagulation and before intraocular surgery:* FA is not routinely indicated in these setting since the low likelihood of significant additional information does not usually justify the additional risk, discomfort and cost to the patient.

- *Post laser:* A must to determine the efficacy of the laser and the requirement for further settings.

References

1. Kaiser N, Sasson S, Feener EP, Differential regulation of glucose transport and transporters by glucose in vascular endothelial and smooth muscle cells, Diabetes, 1993, 42, 80-89.

2. Koya D and King GL, Protein kinase C activation and development of diabetes complications, Diabetes, 1998, 47, 859-866.

3. Derubertis FR and Craven PA, Activation of protein kinase C in glomerular cells in diabetes: Mechanism and potential link to the pathogenesis of diabetic glomerulopathy, Diabetes, 1994, 43, 1-8.

4. Williams B, Glucose-induced vascular smooth muscle dysfunction: the role of protein kinase C, J Hypertens, 1995, 13, 477-486.

5. Baynes JW, Role of oxidative stress in development of complications in diabetes, Diabetes, 1991, 40, 405-412.

6. Jacobs JCR, Das Evcimen N, King GL, New treatments for prevention of insulin resistance and diabetes complications: PKC involvement, 3rd ed., London and New York, Martin Dunitz, 2003.

7. Donnelly R, Protein kinase C: a novel therapeutic target in macrovascular complications, Mod Diabetes Manag, 2000, 1, 13-16.

8. Retina and vitreous (Section 12), The foundation of the American Academy of Ophthalmology, 2000, 88-111.

9. Reqqiero-lopez D, Rellier N, Lecomte M, Wiernspprger N, Growth modulation of retinal microvascular cells by early and advanced glycation product, Diabetes Res Clin Pract, 1997, 34, 135-142.

10. Kowlury RA, Timothy SK, Engerman RL, Abnormalities of retinal metabolism in diabetes or experimental galactosemia IV. Antioxidant defence system, Free red Biol med, 1997, 22, 587-592.

CHAPTER 3

VARIOUS RECEPTORS AND THEIR ACTIVITY IN DIABETIC RETINOPATHY

Receptors and Activity

Mainly three proteins receptors, PKC, VEGF and HIF-1α are responsible for retinopathy and these proteins are interrelated with each other[1]. 12 isomeric forms of PKC receptor are available throughout the body. Differences in their structure and substrate requirements have permitted division of the isomers into three groups shown in **Table 3.1**[2-7].

Table 3.1 Different types of PKC isomers.

Group A	Group B	Group C
Classical	**Novel**	**Atypical**
Calcium dependent	Calcium independent	Calcium independent
Phospholipid dependent	Phospholipid dependent	Phospholipid independent
α	δ	ζ
βI	ε	τ/λ
βII	θ	
γ	η	
	μ	

The PKC Enzyme System

In this system glucose enters the vascular cells by GLUT- I transporter and then metabolized, via glycolysis **(Figure 3.1)**[8]. In patients with

17

diabetes, especially with poor glycemic control, the GLUT-I expression in vascular cells is increased leads to an increase in glycolysis and an increased de-novo synthesis of DAG, which is the main endogenous activator of the PKC system. Studies have shown that in both diabetic animals and humans there is an increase in DAG levels and PKC expression in various tissues, including endothelial, smooth muscle and mesangial cells[9]. The addition or subtraction of phosphate groups is one of the most important mechanisms regulating the activity of cellular proteins: i.e., enzymes and receptors. Major metabolic enzymes such as glycogen synthase are switched on and off by kinases (enzymes that add phosphate groups) and phosphates (enzymes that remove phosphate groups), and these are themselves regulated by other biochemical signals, including hormones and growth factors. There are two different kinds of kinases: those that phosphorylates proteins at tyrosine residue (known as tyrosine kinases), and those that phosphorylates serine and threonine sites (serine/theronine kinases). There are two major serine/threonine kinases widely distributed in all tissues: cyclic-AMP-dependent protein kinase (also known as protein kinase A) and protein kinase C. Increased DAG level in diabetic state can be formed by multiple pathways. DAG can be derived from hydrolysis of phosphatidylinositides, from the metabolism of phosphatidylcholine by phospholipase C- (PLC)[10] or de novo synthesis from glycolytic intermediates, dihydroxyacetone phosphate and glycerol-3-phosphate. De novo synthesis of DAG requires a stepwise acylation catalysed by glycerol-3-phosphate acyltransferase[11]. PKC activation is stimulated by DAG, which contains both saturated and unsaturated fatty acids, including 1-palmitoyl-2-oleoyl-sn-glycerol, although 1-stearoyl- 2-arachidonyl-sn-glycerol may be the most active[12]. DAG-PKC pathway can also be activated by hyperglycemia induced increases in oxidants such as H_2O_2 which are known to activate PKC either directly or by increasing DAG production[13]. In hyperglycemic conditions elevated levels of DAG contained mostly palmitate or oleate fatty acid, supporting the idea that the increased levels of DAG are due to de novo synthesis rather than rapid formation from the actions of phospholipase C.

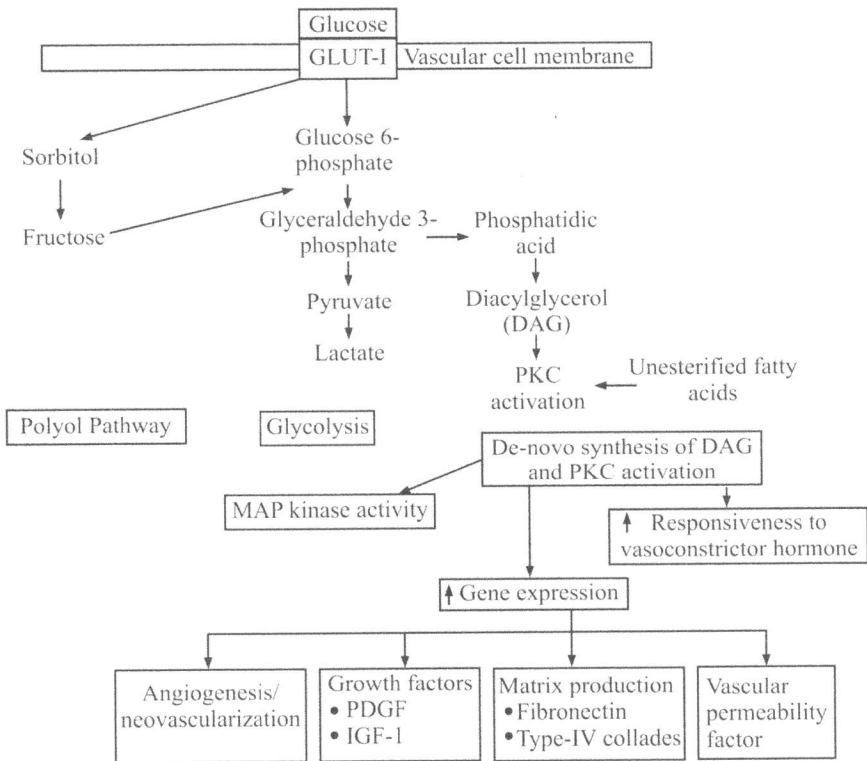

Fig. 3.1 PKC enzyme system and activation of Protein kinase C via glycolysis and PKC action in vascular tissues.

Various PKC Isoforms and There Location in Different Cells

PKC beta II gets activated due to high glucose level in various animal tissues namely brain, aorta, kidney, retina and heart as shown in **Table 3.2**[14-15]. PKC delta is present in brain, heart, spleen, lung, liver, ovary, pancreas, and adrenal tissues. PKC epsilon is present in brain, kidney, and pancreas but predominantly present in brain. PKC zeta is present in most tissues, particularly lungs, brain, and liver. Both PKC delta and PKC zeta showed some heterogeneity of size among the different tissues. PKC alpha is present in all organs and tissues examined but predominantly in brain and spleen. Further, PKC beta I and -beta II are also present in greatest amount in brain and spleen. In case of diabetic retinopathy PKC beta II isoform is more active than other isoforms and PKC beta II isoform is present in high percentage in the retina[16].

Table 3.2 Various PKC isoforms and their location and activation in different cells.

Tissue and cultured cell type	PKC isoforms detected in normal tissue	PKC isoforms activated by high glucose/diabetes
Rat aorta	α, βII	βII
Rat aortic smooth muscle cells	α, βII	βII
	α, βI, βII, δ	βII>δ
Rat Kidney	α, βI, βII, δ, ε, ζ	α, ε
Rat glomeruli	α, βI, βII, δ, ε	α=β
	α, βII, δ, ε	βII
	α, βII, δ, ε	ε>δ>α
Rat mesangial cells	α, δ, ε, ζ	ζ>α
Rat retina	α, βI, βII, ε	βII>ε>α>βI
Bovine retinal endothelial cells	α, βI, βII, δ, ε, ζ	δ>βII>α>βI
Rat corpus cavernosum	α, βI, βII, ε, δ	βII
Rat heart	α, βII	βII
	α, β, δ, ε, ζ	α>δ
	α, β, δ, ε, ζ	A
Rat cardiac monocytes	δ, ε	E
Rat sciatic nerve	α, βI, βII, ε, δ	No difference
	α, βI, βII, ζ	A

Effects of PKC Activation on Various Organs

Multiple diabetic complications have been associated with increased PKC activation. Some of these abnormalities include changes in blood flow, basement membrane thickening, extracellular matrix expansion, vascular permeability, angiogenesis, cell growth and enzymatic activity alterations such as Na^+-K^+-ATPase, $CPLA_2$ and MAP kinase. One of the most prominent features occurring early in diabetes is hemodynamic changes such as changes in blood flow and vascular contractility in many tissues, including the kidney, retina, skin, arteries and nerves.

PKC activation could affect the functions of several vasoactive factors within the kidney. For example, glomerular prostaglandins (PG) E_2, I_2, $F_{2\alpha}$ have been reported to increase after 2 weeks of diabetes[17-18]. Such elevation in PGE_2 and PGI_2 in addition to increased release in arachidonic acid has also been reported in cultured mesangial cells when exposed to elevation of glucose levels. Both elevation and degradation of vasodilator nitric oxide (NO) has been associated with changes of blood flow and contractility leading to glomerular hyperfiltration.

Most studies have demonstrated that PKC activation can decrease retinal blood flow in diabetes mellitus of short duration such as less than 10 years[19-22]. Abnormalities in retinal blood flow and development of retinal ischemia in diabetes can contribute to vessel dysfunction by increasing vascular permeability, enlarging capillary diameter, impairing vascular tone and increasing microaneurism formation. Ischemia of retinal tissues will cause increase in the expression of angiogenic growth factors such as vascular endothelial growth factor (VEGF), leading to macularoedema and proliferative retinopathy[23].

Hyperglycemia induced ischemia has also been suggested to play a role in the development of diabetic neuropathy, since vasodilators, which increase nerve blood flow, appear to improve nerve function in diabetic rodents[24]. However, a role for PKC activation in diabetic neuropathy is not clear, since some reports have suggested that PI (phosphatidyl inositol) turnover and DAG levels were reduced[25] and cause a decreased in PKC activity in the peripheral nerves. Diminished PKC activity may reduce the Na^+-K^+-ATPase phosphorylation leading to a decrease in nerve conduction and nerve regeneration.

PKC activation can directly increase permeability of macromolecules[26] across the endothelial or epithelial barriers by phosphorylating cytoskeletal proteins[27] or by regulating expression or activity of various growth factors[28]. PKC activation has been reported to phosphorylate cytoskeletal proteins caldesmon, vimentin, talin and vinculin. Overexpression of PKCβ1 in human dermal microvascular endothelial cells was reported to enhance phorbol ester-induced effects to increase permeability to albumin.

VEGF Receptors

VEGF are important signaling proteins involved in vasculogenesis and angiogenesis. Currently, the VEGF family consists of seven members, VEGF A, VEGF B, VEGF C, VEGF D, VEGF E, VEGF F, and P1GF with distinct individual monomeric forms consisting of 121, 145, 165, 183, 189, and 206 amino acids respectively. These VEGF isomers act via three specific tyrosin kinase receptors- VEGFR1/Flt-1, VEGFR2/Flk-1, and VEGFR3/Flt-4[29]. The detailed function of each receptor has not been completely determined however these VEGFRs have been targeted due to their role in angiogenesis. Increased concentration of VEGF in various organs causes serious pathological conditions like cerebral venous infarcts and vasogenicoedema in brain, retinal/choroidal neovascularization and macularoedema in eyes, and increased glomerular permeability in kidney. Where as decrease in VEGF level also causes various pathological conditions like stroke and impaired reparative neurogenesis in brain, impaired development of collateral vessels in heart, vascular hypertension, collapse of capillary loops and impaired podocyte function in kidney, neuropathy and impairement of wound healing[30]. **Table 3.3** describes the biochemical changes due to impaired activity of VEGF receptors.

Table 3.3 VEGF receptor role in VEGF regulated and activated conditions.

Receptor	Role	Locations	Activation associated with pathology
VEGF-R1 (Flt-1)	Acts as decoy, sequestering VEGF, regulating VEGF/VEGF-R2 interaction, involved in angiogenesis and vasculogenesis.	Membrane bound. Expressed in endothelial, macrophage-lineage cells, neurons and glial cells.	Tumor growth, metastasis, inflammation, rheumatoid arthritis, artherosclorosis.
VEGF-R2 (Flk-1)	Regulates fenestrations and permeability in eye and kidney. Directly transmits signals associated with pathological angiogenesis. Involved in vasculogenesis and endothelial progenitor cell recruitment.	Membrane bound. Abundant in vascular or lymphatic epithelial cells.	Cancer, diabetic retinopathy and other diseases with pathological angiogenesis and hypertension.
VEGF-R3	Key to wound healing by activating VEGF-C and VEGF-D	Membrane bound.	Metastasis of cancer to the lymph nodes
sFlt-1 (soluble VEGF-R1)	"Soaks up" available VEGF, prevents vascularization in the cornea. Regulates angiogenesis.	Non-membrane bound. Present in serum and tissue.	Metastasis of cancer to the lymph nodes, pre-eclampsia, hypertension, proteinuria, renal dysfunction, preventing ocular vascularization.

VEGF and Diabetic Retinopathy

VEGF is produced by several types of cells within the eye (retinal pigment epithelial cells, glial cells, retinal capillary pericytes, endothelial cells, Mullar cells and ganglion cells) and is a critical stimulus for DME and both retinal and choroidal neovascularization. Diabetic patients PDR or DME have elevated intraocular VEGF in the vitreous and aqueous fluids that are correlated with disease presence and severity. It should be noted that the vitreal levels detected in PDR patients are in the range of those that induce neovascularization *in vitro*. In consequence, vitreous accumulation of VEGF derived from widespread production of this factor by ischemic retina contributes significantly to the intraocular neovascularization. Apart from higher intraocular VEGF concentrations, a two-fold increase in VEGF receptor expression has been reported in the retinas from diabetic rats. Systemic VEGF is also related to retinal pathology: plasma VEGF is elevated in patients with hypertension and retinopathy compared with controls and related to retinopathy severity in Type 1 diabetics.

The mechanism by which VEGF indues neovascularisation in PDR are multifactorial. The increase of VEGF induced by hypoxia and AGEs, as well as the enhancement of VEGF receptors, will be crucial in determining its angiogenic effect. The signaling pathways induced by the activation of VEGF receptors. Apart from its mitogenic effect, VEGF favors the proteolysis of basement membrane, which is the first step in the angiogenic process that leads to PDR. Another mechanism by which VEGF could promote angiogenesis is though the enhancement of vascular adhesion molecule 1 (VCAM-1). In this regard, a direct correlation between VCAM-1 and VEGF in the vitreous fluid of PDR patients has been reported. In recent years, an anti-angiogenic family of VEGF isoforms has been discovered and termed VEGF (xxx) b, where xxx is the number of amino acids encoded. VEGF (xxx) b isoforms aries from an alternative 3′ splice site in exon 8, and differ by a mere six amino acids at the C-terminus. These alternative six amino acids radically change the functional properties of VEGF. The first member of this family to be identified was $VEGF_{165}b$; it is the only form which has been characterized in terms of its action on endothelial cells. A single injection of $VEGF_{165}b$ can significantly reduce preretinal neovascularization without inhibition of physiology intraretinal angiogenesis in the oxygen induced retinopathy mouse model of ocular neovascularization. DR is associated with a switch in splicing from anti-to-pro-angiogenic isoforms of VEGF. Therefore, the understanding of what regulates VEGF (xxx) b alternative splicing, and consequently, the balance of pro-and anti-angiogenic isoforms is of great importance and may provide a novel therapeutic strategy for PDR and DME. Intraocular sFlt-1 levels are also associated with diabetic ocular disease. Elevated intraocular VEGF and reduced intraocular sFlt-1 levels have been found in PDR diabetic patients in comparision with patients with macular holes. Since sFlt-1 supressess VEGF-induced retinal vascular permeability in experimental models, reduced sFlt-1 in patients with PDR may foster VEGF-instigated angiogenesis. In addition, gene transfer of sFlt-1 via periocular injections reduced choroidal neovascularization in mice.

Intracellular Relationship between VEGF and PKC

PKC is a signal transducer which activates or inhibits VEGF and VEGF in turn activates or inhibit PKC. Therefore, PKC and VEGF form a vicious cycle in an intracellular process of biochemical pathophysiology of neovascularization **(Figure 3.2).** Since PKC family is widely distributed through out the body and the inhibition of PKC isoforms would also suppress VEGF.

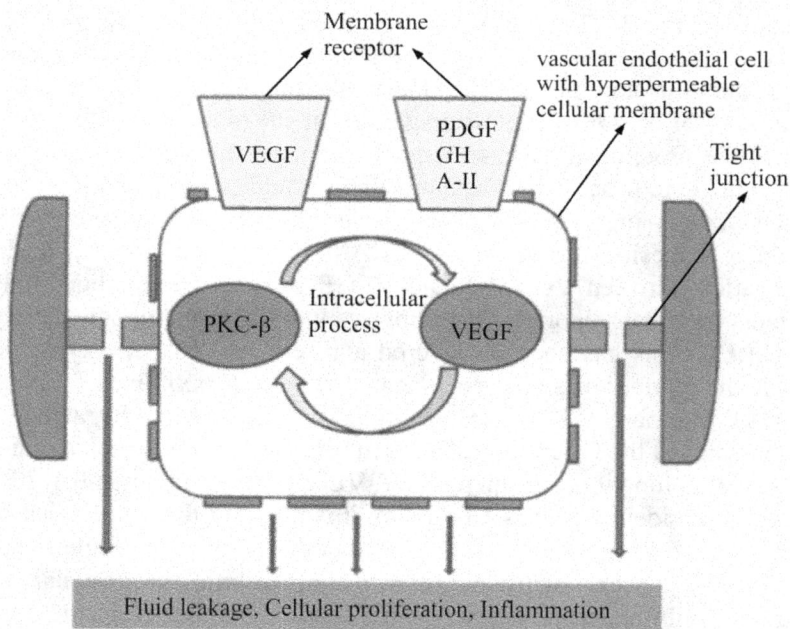

Fig. 3.2 Intracellular relationship between PKC and VEGF.

Angiogenesis and Retinopathy

In healthy adults, the vasculature is quiescent except during wound healing, hair growth and the menstrual cycle. Otherwise, endothelial cells show very little proliferation. Imbalance in the demand and supply of oxygen and nutrients, as occur in the course of, for instance, proliferative diabetic retinopathy, tumor growth, or myocardial infraction, results in sprouting of new capillaries from pre-existing vessels, a process called angiogenesis. Local growth of vessels is induced by the release of soluble angiogenic factors by the tissues involved, which activate endothelial cells. Interactions of angiogenic factors with their receptors by the tissue involved, which activate endothelial cells. Interactions of angiogenic factors with their receptors provide signals for cell migration, proliferation and differentiation to form new capillaries [31].

Angiogenesis is a complex process, characterized by a cascade of events: initial vasodilation of existing vessels is accompanied by increased vascular permeability and degradation of the surrounding matrix, which allows activated and proliferating endothelial cells to migrate and form tubes. These endothelial cells of sprouting vessels are thought to be supported by a network of differentiated pre-endothelial cells and matrix. Subsequently, a phase of maturation and remodeling of these new vessels takes place to form a vascular network.

Mechanism of Angiogenesis: The regulation of angiogenesis by hypoxia is probably mediated by a key transcriptional regulator, hypoxia-inducible factor (HIF-1), a hetero dimer (α and β subunits), first recognized as a DNA-binding factor that mediates the hypoxia-inducible activity of the erythropoietin. HIF-1 stimulates angiogenesis by activating transcription of the gene for VEGF and there is a correlation between expression of HIF-1 and tumor grade and vascularization in brain, breast and other common human tumors. Increased levels of HIF-1 α have been reported in the ischemic retina in the mouse model of retinopathy and this has a temporal and spatial correlation with increased expression of VEGF [32]. Hypoxia causes upregulation of growth factors most of which then stimulate endothelial cell proliferation. Growth factors can also cause increasd expression of integrins and proteinases both of which are important for cell migration. Both endothelial cell proliferation and migration are important key steps in angiogenesis **(Figure 3.3)**. The switch to the angiogenic step depends on a balance between angiogenic factors and endogenous angiogenesis inhibitors.

Capillary Nonperfusion
(Increase Platelet aggregation, Leukocyte adhesion, ICAM and decrease Prostacyclin)

```
                    ┌─────────┐      ┌──────────┐
                    │  HIF-1  │◄─────│ HYPOXIA  │
                    └─────────┘      └──────────┘
```

Increase VEGF, Flt-1, ICF-1,
Ang2   Growth Factor

Integrins   Integrins
(Increase avb3 and avb5)   Lysis of ECM & BM (Increase MMp-2,
                                                MMp-9, Urokinase)

CELL MIGRATION   CELL PROLIFERATION

ANGIOGENESIS

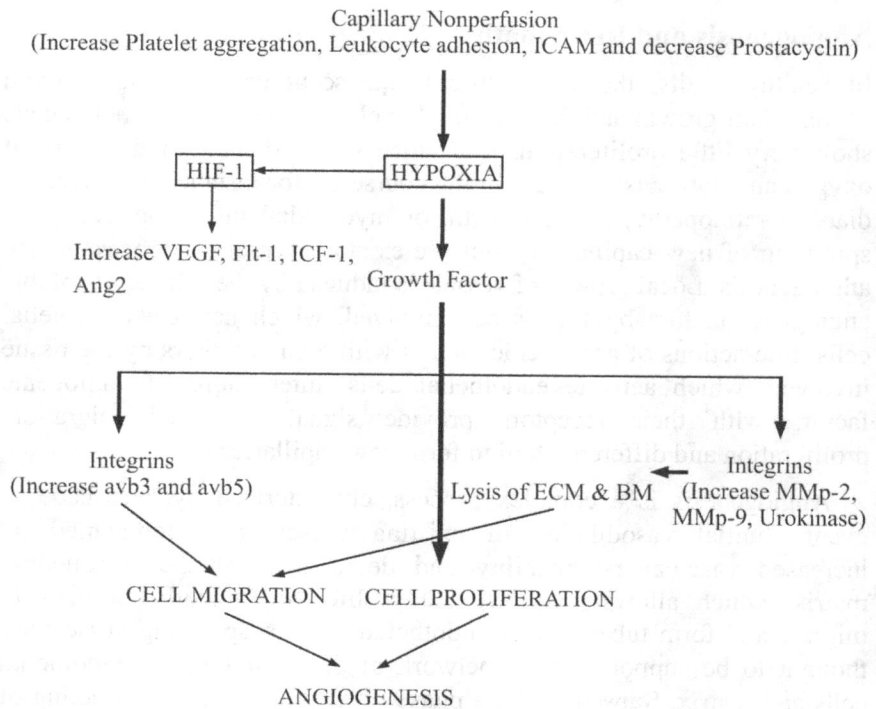

Fig. 3.3 Mechanism of retinal angiogenesis.

For the analysis of anti-angiogenic activity various *in-vitro* and *in-vivo* studies are available shown in **Table 3.4.**

Table 3.4 *In-vitro* and *in-vivo* angiogenesis assays

Assay	Measurement	Comments
Cell Proliferation	Inhibition of cell doubling opposing stimulatory effect of a defined angiogenic factor	Cytostatic activity blocks cell proliferation without causing cell death
Cell migration	Inhibition of cell migration opposing stimulatory effect of a defined angiogenic factor such as VEGF or bFGF	The extension of endothelial cell processes allows cells to migrate over a substratum
Invasion	Inhibition of cell invasion opposing stimulatory effect of a defined angiogenic factor	The growth of endothelial cells through a porous membrane or matrix in response to a chemotactic factor

Table 4 *Contd...*

Assay	Measurement	Comments
Sprouting	Inhibition of migration, invasion and tube formation in a 3D matrix of collagen I or fibrin opposing stimulatory effect of a defined angiogenic factor	An integrated assay which couples vascular invasion, tube formation and maturation in 3D matrix
Matrigel cord assay	Inhibition of cord assembly by endothelial cells on complex matrix derived from tumor stroma opposing stimulatory effect of a defined angiogenic factor	Endothelial cells assembly into cords over the matrix
Chorioallantoic Mambrane (CAM) *in vivo*	Inhibition of blood vessels growth in the CAM of a fertilized developing chicken egg	The developing vasculature of the CAM is highly sensitive inhibitors of angiogenesis
Corneal angiogenesis *in-vivo*	Inhibition of de novo capillary growth in cornea opposing stimulatory effect of a defined angiogenic factor	Blood vessels from surrounding sclera vessel supply invade the avascular cornea in response to slow-release growth factor implanted in cornea
Matrigel *in vivo*	Inhibition of blood vessel growth into a matrigel plug implanted in abdominal region of mouse	Blood vessels invade the Matrigel plug in response to stimulus from growth factor impregnated plug

References

1. George LK and Evcimen ND, The role of protein kinase C activation and the vascular complications of diabetes, Pharmacol Res, 2007, 55, 498-510.

2. Nishizuka Y, Intracellular signaling by hydrolysis of phospholipids and activation of protein kinase C, Science, 258, 607-614.

3. Hotmann J, The potential for isoenzymes-selective modulation of protein kinase C, FASEB J, 11, 649-669.

4. Kanashiro CA and Khalil RA, Signal transduction by protein kinase C in mammalian cells, Clin Exp Physiol Pharmacol, 25, 974-985.

5. Liu WS and Heckman CA, The sevenfold way of PKC regulation, Cell Signal, 10, 529-542.

6. Mellor H and Parker PJ, The extended protein kinase C superfamily, Biochem J, 332, 281-292.

7. Newton AC, Regulation of protein kinase C, Curr Opin Cell Biol, 9, 161-167.

8. Donnelly R, Protein kinase C: a novel therapeutic target in macrovascular complications, Mod Dia Manag, 2000, 1, 13-16.

9. King GL, The role of hyperglycemia and hyperinsulinaemia in causing vascular dysfunction in diabetes, Annals of Med, 1996, 28, 427-432.

10. Nishizuka Y, Intracellular signaling by hydrolysis of phospholipids and activation of protein kinase C, Science, 1992, 258, 607-614.

11. Berne C, The metabolism of lipids in mouse pancreatic islets. The biosynthesis of triacylglycerols and phospholipids, Biochem J, 1975, 152, 667-673.

12. Sekiguchi GM, Nomura K, Kikkawa HN, Nishizuka Y, Further studies on the specificity of diacylglycerol for protein kinase C activation, Biochem Biophys Res Commun, 1985, 132, 467-473.

13. Konishi H, Tanaka M, Takemura Y, Matsuzaki H, Ono Y, Kikkawa U, Activation of protein kinase C by tyrosine phosphorylation in response to H_2O_2, Proc Natl Acad Sci, 1997, 94, 11233-11237.

14. Hofmann J, The potential for isoenzymes-selective modulation of protein kinase C, FASEB J, 1997, 11, 649-669.

15. Mellor H and Parker PJ, The extende protein kinase C superfamily, Biochem J, 1998, 332, 281-292.

16. William CW, Khan WA, Merchenthaler I, Tissue and Cellular Distribution of the Extended Family of Protein Kinase C Isoenzymes, J Chem Biol, 1992, 117, 121-133.

17. Schambelan M, Blake S, Sraer J, Bens M, Nives MP, Wahbe F, Increased prostaglandin production by glomeruli isolated from rats with streptozotocin-induced diabetes mellitus, J Clin Invest, 1985, 75, 404-412.

18. Craven PA, Caines MA, DeRubertis FR, Sequential alterations in glomerular prostaglandin and thromboxane synthesis in diabetic rats: relationship to the hyperfiltration of early diabetes, metabolism, J Clin Invest, 1987, 36, 95-103.

19. Feke GT, Buzney SM, Ogasawara H, Fujio N, Goger DG, Spack NP, Retinal circulatory abnormalities in type I diabetes, Invest Ophthalmol Vis Sci, 1994, 35, 2968-2975.

20. Bursell SE, Clermont AC, Kinsley BT, Simonson DC, Aiello LM, Wolpert HA, Retinal blood flow changes in patients with insulin-dependent diabetes mellitus and no diabetic retinopathy, Invest Ophthalmol Vis Sci, 1996, 37, 886-897.

21. Small KW, Stefansson E, Hatchell D, Retinal blood flow in normal and diabetic dogs, Invest Ophthalmol Vis Sci, 1987, 28, 672-675.

22. Miyamoto K, Ogura Y, Nishiwaki H, Matsuda N, Honda Y, Kato S, Evaluation of retinal microcirculatory alterations in the Goto-Kakizaki rat, Invest Ophthalmol Vis Sci, 1996, 37, 898-905.

23. Aiello LP, Avery RI, Arrigg PG, Keyt BA, Jampel HD, Shah ST, Vascular endothelial growth factor in ocular fluid of patients with diabetic retinopathy and other retinal disorders, N Engl J Med, 1994, 331, 1480-1487.

24. Cameron NE and Cotter MA, Metabolic and vascular factors in the pathogenesis of diabetic neuropathy, Diabetes, 1997, 46, S31-S37.

25. Uehara K, Yamagishi S, Otsuki S, Chin S, Yagihashi S, Effects of polyol pathway hyperactivity on protein kinase C activity, nociceptive peptide expression and neuronal structure in dorsal root ganglia in diabetic mice, Diabetes, 2004, 53, 3239-3247.

26. Lynch JJ, Ferro TJ, Blumenstock FA, Brockenauer AM, Malik AB, Increased endothelial albumin permeability mediated by protein kinase C activation, J Clin Invest, 1990, 85, 1991-1998.

27. Wolf BA, Williamson JR, Easom RA, Chang K, Sherman WR, Turk J, Diacylglycerol accumulation and microvascular abnormalities induced by elevated glucose levels, J Clin Invest, 1991, 87, 31-38.

28. Katsura Y, Okano T, Noritake M, Kosano H, Nishigori H, Kado S, Hepatocyte growth factor in vitreous fluid of patients with proliferative diabetic retinopathy and other retinal disorders, Dia Care, 1998, 21, 1759-1763.

29. Ferrata N, Gerber HP, LeCouter J, The biology of VEGF and its receptors, Nat Med, 2003, 9, 669-676.

30. Wirostko B, Wong TY, Simo R, Vascular endothelial growth factor and diabetic complicatins, Prog in Retinal and Eye Res, 2008, 27, 608-621.

31. Ferrara N, Chen H, Davis-Smyth T, Gerber HP, Nguyen TN, Peers D, Chisholm V, Hillan KJ, Schwall RH, Vascular endothelial growth factor is essential for corpus luteum angiogenesis, Nat Med, 2007, 4, 336-340.

32. Ozaki H, Yu AY, Della K, Ozaki K, Luna JD, Yamada H, Hackett SF, Okamoto N, Zack DJ, Semenza GL, Campochiaro PA, Hypoxia inducible factor-1 alpha is increased in ischemic retina: temporal and spatial correlation with VEGF expression, Invest Ophtalmology Vis Sci, 2002, 40, 182-189.

CHAPTER 4

AVAILABLE CURRENT
TREATMENTS

In general laser photocoagulation surgery is advised for patients with high risk PDR and for patients with CSME, since both groups have better visual prognosis when treated.

Photocoagulation

The cornerstone of the management of diabetic retinopathy is photocoagulation. It is a therapeutic technique employing a strong light source to coagulate tissue. Light energy is absorbed by the target tissue and converted into thermal energy. When tissue temperature rises above 65°C, denaturation of tissue proteins and coagulative necrosis occur. Most surgeons perform photocoagulation with lasers spanning the visible light spectrum of 400 to 780 nm. The presently favoured laser in this spectrum is the frequency-doubled Nd-Yag system apart from the time-honoured argon blue-green. Diode laser with 810 nm is also in vogue[1-2].

Delivery systems may employ a transpupillary approach with slit lamp delivery, indirect ophthalmoscopic application, endophotocoagulation during vitrectomy surgery and trans-scleral application with a contact probe. Selection of laser setting parameters depends on the intent of treatment, the clarity of ocular media and the fundus pigmentation. As a general rule, smaller spot sizes require lesser energy than larger spot sizes, and longer duration exposures require less energy than short duration exposures to achieve the same intensity effect.

Laser is applied in the form of spots. When it is applied in a localized area, it is known as focal laser, as would happen when laser is applied to a leaking area in the macular area clinically seen as a circinate ring of HE. When laser spots are applied over the entire retinal area visualized, it is termed as panretinal photocoagulation or scatter laser photo-coagulation.

The basic rationale of photocoagulation is to destroy neovascular complexes, to obliterate areas of microinfraction or capillary closure, to destroy leaking vessels in the macular or paramacular area and ultimately produce chorioretinal vitreoretinal traction. The proliferation of new vessels is provable a result of localized hypoxia in the region of retinal vessels near the internal limiting membrane. It would seem obvious that these blood vessels are proliferating in response to some biochemical stimulus and neovascularization appears to be an appropriate defence for the preparative mechanism of the body. However, the in-growth of the neovascularization with support of the glial tissue, as well as the attendant leakage of damaged vessels into the surrounding retinal spaces, the transport of high molecular weight lipoproteinaceous material through the neovascular walls into the retina, the resulting haemorrhages and the dynamic changes occurring from interposition of fibrovascular membranes can irreversibly damage the macular retina.

Panretinal photocoagulation (PRP) appears to successfully obliterate or cause the regression of neovascularization by one of the four mechanisms:

(a) The reduction or destruction of hypoxic retina that is producing the vasoformative factor (could be vascular endothelial growth factor) that is calling forth neovascularization from more healthy areas of the retina.

(b) The creation of closer opposition of the inner layers of the retina to the choriocapillaries by multiple scattered photocoagulation scarring around the entire posterior polar region, thereby allowing greater oxygen perfusion from the choroidal layers to the inner retinal layers that have undergone a relatively high degree of microinfracted areas of retina and slugging perfused capillaries, thereby allowing the blood to increase the nourishment of the remaining retina.

(c) The destruction of leaking blood vessels and other abnormal vascular complexes that are creating abnormal haemodynamic situation in the diabetic retina, thereby more nearly normalizing the vascular supply of the macular region of the eye.

The entire concept of the vasoformative factor being elaborated by the hypoxic retina, secondary to microinfraction and capillary closure, is a most inviting explanation for the beneficial effects of PRP. If, the vasoformative factor emanating from the hypoxic areas of the retina can be reduced in the posterior vitreous, the neovascular stimulus is thereby decreased, and the new vessels tend to regress or become obliterated. Certainly the better nutrition of the inner portions of the retina by closer opposition of the inner layers to the choriocapillaries and the choroidal blood supply would also appear to be a beneficial result of the PRP technique.

Focal laser in the macular area is termed as a grid laser. Usually this grid is applied in the form of a reserve C with the arms of the C starting at the origin of the arcades beyond the papillomacular bundle. Upon angiographic evaluation, selective grid laser can be done around a leaking site in the macular area.

PRP of one eye is usually applied in two-three settings. If focal macular laser is to be done along with PRP, it is usually done with the first setting of PRP. PDR is treated with PRP and CSME with focal laser photocoagulation. Some patients with high risk PDR or with severe or very severe NPDR may also benefit from PRP depending upon such factors as: diabetes type, medical status, access to care, compliance with follow-up, status and progression of fellow eye, family history, neovacularization of the angle and iris is also indication of PRP.

Limiation of Laser Therapy

Laser surgery and vitrectomy are very successful, but they donot cure diabetic retinopathy. Laser treatment can be painful; it permanantly damages the retina and is often ineffective on the medium or long term. It slightly reduces preipharal vision, change colour perception and impairs night vision due to loss of retinal tissue. In case of proliferative diabetic retinopathy, always be at risk for new bleeding. Therefore, there is an urgent need for the development of new therapies to prevent and treat DR[3].

Evidence-Based Options for the Medical Treatment of Diabetic Retinopathy

Diabetic Retinopathy and Blood Glucose Control

Tight control of glycemia reduces the risk of onset and progression of DR, similar to that observed for other microvascular complications. This was conclusively demonstrated by 2 major intervention studies, the DCCT[4], performed on patients with T1DM, and the United Kingdom Prospective Diabetes Study[5], carried out on newly diagnosed people with T2DM.

The DCCT included 1441 patients, 726 with no DR and 715 with mild DR, who was followed up for an average 6.5 years. The trial aimed at comparing intensive versus conventional insulin treatment in the primary and secondary prevention of DR. To be included, the patients must be neither hypertensive nor hypercholesterolemic or prone to severe hypoglycemia. Intensive insulin treatment meant at least 3 daily injections or continuous subcutaneous infusion with dosages adjusted according to minimum 4-daily self monitoring, monthly visits in clinic, and medical, dietary, educational, and psychological support available over 24 hr. The goals were fasting blood glucose between 70 and 120 mg/dL (3.9 and 6.7 mmol/L), postprandial glucose below 180 mg/dL (10 mmol/L), and glycosylated hemoglobin (HbA1c) within the reference range (66.05%). Conventional therapy meant 1–2 daily injections without adjusting the doses, self-monitoring of blood or urine, 3 monthly appointments, and generic education on treatment, diet, and exercise. The targets were to remain free of ketonuria and symptoms and maintain stable growth and body weight. During follow-up, patients on intensive treatment maintained an average HbA1c of 7.2%, versus 9.1% for those on conventional therapy. Intensified treatment reduced the onset of new retinopathy by 76%, the risk of existing DR worsening by 54%, the progression to severe nonproliferative diabetic retinopathy by 47%, and the need for photocoagulation by 56%. Extrapolation of these results over lifetime suggests that intensive treatment can buy patients 14.7 more years free from PDR, 8.2 free from CSME, and 7.7 free from blindness[6]. On the down side, intensified insulin treatment caused 3 times as many severe hypoglycemic episodes and a 33% increased risk of becoming overweight. Seven years later, when all DCCT patients had returned to their habitual care, differences in metabolic control were abolished, but those who had been on intensive treatment maintained their advantage in terms of reduced risks of worsening of DR and need for photo-coagulation[7], suggesting that years of good control remain stored in some kind of metabolic memory, as far as tissue complications are concerned. Interestingly, it took 20 years for patients under strict glycemic control to reach a statistically significant benefit over those under conventional treatment. In fact, during the first year of intensified insulin delivery, about 10% of patients who already had moderate to severe NPDR experienced worsening of their lesions, called early worsening phenomenon. The UKPDS enrolled 3867 newly diagnosed T2DM patients aged 48–60 who, after 3 months on diet only, were randomized to intensive treatment with either sulfonylureas or insulin (the target being fasting blood glucose 66 mmol/L [108 mg/dL]) or conventional policy (i.e., the best fasting blood glucose achievable by diet alone, with drugs added only if levels went above 15 mmol/L [270 mg/dL] or symptoms appeared). Eye-related end points included blindness (visual acuity b6/60) in 1 eye, 2-step worsening of DR on the ETDRS scale, based upon 7-field stereo color photographs, 3-line worsening of visual acuity on the logMAR chart (doubling of the visual angle), and an aggregate microvascular end point including onset of vitreous hemorrhage, need for photocoagulation, and cataract extraction. Maintaining HbA1c lower by 0.9% over 12 years reduced the risk of DR worsening by 21%, the need for photocoagulation by 29%, and cataract extraction by 24%. Nonsignificant reductions were observed for vitreous hemorrhages and blindness in 1 eye. Like in the DCCT, also in the UKPDS, intensified treatment caused weight gain (on average 3.1 kg) and increased risk for hypoglycemia.

The Early Worsening Phenomenon

As observed in the DCCT and some previous trials on the effects of intensified treatment on retinopathy, some patients experience the early worsening phenomenon (i.e., temporary worsening of preexisting retinopathy of mild to moderate severity). This is not a constant or predictable occurrence and may affect up to one third of patients undergoing rapid improvement of glycemic control. Worsening occurs during the first 6–12 months, after which retinopathy tends to stabilize and, within 2 years, will take a slower rate of progression compared with patients remaining on conventional treatment. A practical consequence is that, before optimizing glycemic control, the presence and severity of DR should be verified. Sometimes, photocoagulation might have to be considered. The mechanisms through which a rapid reduction of glycemia leads to worsening of retinopathy are not clear. A widely held hypothesis is that lowering blood glucose reduces retinal blood flow and, since DR is mostly the consequence of retinal ischemia due to progressive capillary closure, this would cause further hypoxia. In experimental animals, increasing blood glucose from 15 to 55 mmol/L increases retinal blood flow by about 20%[8]. However, direct measurements of retinal blood flow by laser Doppler velocimetry suggested that the opposite may be true, as retinal flow increased in the patient's inwhom DR worsened after improvement of metabolic control. These results were interpreted as possible evidence for a pathogenetic role of increasing shear stress on the vessel wall[9]. Finally, a third hypothesis put forward by Chantelau and Kohner[10] suggested that enhanced hepatic insulinization may increase the production of insulin-like growth factor 1 (IGF-1), thus facilitating angiogenesis either directly or by potentiating the activity of vascular endothelial growth factor (VEGF) expressed in the retina[11].

Diabetic retinopathy and hypertension

Between 38% and 68% of people with T2DM are also affected by hypertension[12]. Although observational studies did not agree in considering it as an independent risk factor, a substudy of the UKPDS demonstrated that strict control of blood pressure is effective in reducing the progression of retinopathy and loss of vision. The study population included 1148 patients affected by T2DM and hypertension, and the aims were to establish if stricter blood pressure control would reduce the morbidity and mortality associated with diabetes and whether a particular drug class (angiotensin-converting enzyme (ACE) inhibitor or h-blockers) would show specific advantages in terms of efficacy and prevention of vascular complications. The patients were randomized to receive either treatment according to a less strict (180/105 mmHg) or stricter blood pressure target (150/85 mmHg).

After 9 years of treatment, captopril and atenolol were equally effective in reducing blood pressure, 144/83 and 143/81 mmHg, respectively; although diastolic values were significant lower among patients allocated to the β-blocker. The risk of a 2-step worsening of DR was reduced by 24% after 6 years and by 34% after 9 years and the observation that the ACE inhibitor and the β-blocker were equally effective suggests that this result was due to lowering blood pressure rather than drug-specific mechanisms. Hypertension might contribute to worsening of DR by increasing endothelial shear stress and the release of VEGF that follows stretching of the vessel walls[13], leading to altered retinal autoregulation and increased perfusion pressure[14]. The target blood pressure of 130/85 mmHg, which is recommended for the management of patients with diabetes, particularly those with microalbuminuria, is certainly lower than the levels that proved effective in the UKPDS and would presumably prove effective also in the prevention of DR. Although β-blockers and thiazide diuretics may worsen glycemic control by altering insulin secretion and decreasing its peripheral action[15], this effect is minor in clinical termsand more than offset by the proven advantages of these drugs in reducing cardiovascular morbidity and mortality associated with hypertension[16]. ACE inhibitors, on the other hand, may improve glycemic control, promote the differentiation of adipocytes, and improve insulin sensitivity and muscular blood flow. No data are available for angiotension receptor blockers.

Inhibition of the renin-angiotensin system

There is *in vitro* evidence that angiotensin II increases glucose uptake by retinal pericytes[17], induces the release of VEGF by retinal endothelial cells, and that blockade of the reninangiotensin system may prevent new vessel growth in a transgenic animal model of retinopathy of prematurity. In experimental animals, lisinopril reduces VEGF levels and the expression of VEGF receptors independently of blood pressure. Retinal storage of glucose was reduced by 48% in rats treated with captopril, whereas atenolol had no such effect[18]. ACE inhibitors act by inhibiting angiotensin II synthesis, but there are alternative pathways to angiotension II production, which are not blocked by these drugs. Studies focused on angiotensin I receptor blockers have shown that losartan reduces leukocyte entrapment in retinal vessels of rats and that candesartan reduces VEGF and ameliorates retinal abnormalities in diabetic rats[19]. Such observations suggest that inhibition of the reninangiotensin system in the eye may have useful effects in the prevention of DR that are independent of blood pressure reduction. On the clinical side, EURODIAB Controlled Trial of Lisinopril in Insulin-Dependent Diabetes Mellitus (EUCLID), a randomized trial, reported that lisinopril reduced DR progression by 50% and development of PDR by 80% over 2 years in normotensive patients with T1DM with a drop of only 3 mmHg in systolic blood pressure[20]. However, DR was not a primary outcome of EUCLID, the sample was undersized, there were some confounding factors, and other trials, such as the Heart Outcomes Prevention Evaluation (2000) and the Appropriate Blood Pressure Control in Diabetes Trial, which also included DR among their secondary end points, do not support the notion that ACE inhibitors have specific effects on the course of retinopathy. The Diabetic Retinopathy Candesartan Trials, a clinical trial appropriately targeted and powered, is of course to find out whether candesartan is effective in the primary and secondary prevention of retinopathy in patients with T1DM and in the secondary prevention in patients with T2DM[21].

Anti-aggregating agents

Multiple occlusions of retinal capillaries are considered a critical step in the development of DR. Increased platelet aggregation was suggested to contribute to the pathogenesis of DR[22], and early observational studies had suggested that patients on chronic aspirin treatment because of rheumatoid arthritis may be less prone to retinopathy. The use of high doses of aspirin also decreased leukocyte adhesion to retinal capillaries, arteries, and veins in diabetic subjects, reduced integrin expression on the surface of leukocytes and the presence of adhesion molecules (intercellular adhesion molecule 1) on the capillary wall[23]. Again, when the matter was brought to clinical test, a large trial showed minimal effects of aspirin and ticlopidine in reducing the progression of mild DR, and the ETDRS conclusively showed that aspirin has no effect on the progression of severe DR, except it does not increase the risk of bleeding from new vessels in patients with PDR. Hence, PDR is not a contraindication to anti-aggregating treatment for the prevention of cardiovascular events.

Growth hormone inhibitors

The role of growth hormone (GH) and IGF-1 in the pathogenesis of DR is supported by the new-historical clinical observation of regression of severe proliferative retinopathy in a patient who developed postpartum pituitary apoplexy. Clinical studies have often demonstrated increased release of GH and IGF-1 in diabetic patients with DR, and in vitro data showed that GH stimulates the proliferation of human retinal endothelial cells. The role of IGF-1 in the pathogenesis of DR is controversial. Some authors have proposed a vasoprotective effect for this mediator of GH[24], which, on the other hand, may also play a permissive role in the process leading to neovascularization. A role for somatostatin in retinal homeostasis is supported by the observation that levels of somatostatin like immunoreactivity in patients with diabetes is lower in the vitreous than in the plasma[25]. Inhibiting GH production by octreotide, a long-acting analogue of somatostatin was reported to reduce the progression of severe DR. A randomized, double-blind, controlled clinical trial is currently being carried out in patients with severe NPDR.

Protein kinase C inhibitors

Hyperglycemia leads to persistent de novo synthesis and activation of protein kinase C (PKC), induced by increased glucose availability through diacyglycerol (DAG) which, in turn, is associated with a number of biochemical and metabolic abnormalities[26]. The PKC-beta and PKC-y isoforms predominate in the vascular tissue and the former, in particular, plays an important role in modulating the production of VEGF/vascular permeability factor, thus affecting growth and permeability of the retinal endothelium. A selective inhibitor of PKC-, βII ruboxistaurin mesylate (LY333531), is being tested for its potentially beneficial effects on moderate to severe DR. Preliminary results suggest that ruboxistaurin might reduce macular edema in eyes with DR[27] (Table 4.1).

Table 4.1 Inhibitors of classical PKCs in clinical trials.

Name	status	specificity	Binding site
Enzastaurin (LY-317615)	Phase III	PKCβ	ATP-binding site competitive
Ruboxistaurin (LY-333531)	Phase III	PKCβ	ATP-binding site competitive
Midostaurin (PKC421)	Phase II	PKC FLT3 VEGFR2 Kit PDGFR	ATP-binding site competitive
UCN-01 (KW-2401, NSC-638850)	Phase II DISCONTINUED	PKCs CDKs PDK1 Chk1/2	ATP-binding site competitive
Lestaurtinib (CEP-701, KT-5555)	Phase III	PKCs FLT3 TrkA	ATP-binding site competitive
Ro-31-8220	Pre-clinical	PKC	ATP-binding site competitive
Gö6976	Pre-clinical	c PKC	ATP-binding site competitive
Bryostatin-1	Phase II DISCONTINUED	PKC	Regulatory domain
Safingol (SPC-100270)	Phase I DISCONTINUED	PKC	Regulatory domain
Aprinocarsen (LY-900003), Affinitak ISIS-3521	Phase III DISCONTINUED	PKCα	mRNA

Other Therapies

Knowledge of the mechanisms through which hyperglycemia causes the chronic complications of diabetes would provide a basis upon which to plan preventive and therapeutic strategies. Apart from the approaches that are currently undergoing phase 3 trials, mechanisms suspected of producing cell damage in diabetes and which present a potential for pharmacological correction include polyol pathway activation leading to sorbitol accumulation, production of advanced glycation end products (AGE), blood lipids, leukocyte adhesion to the vessel wall, inappropriate angiogenesis, and increased oxidative stress.

Aldose reductase inhibitors: Chronic hyperglycemia increases the metabolic flux through the polyol pathway, leading to the conversion of glucose into sorbitol through the key enzyme aldose reductase, decreasing intracellular concentrations of NADPH, reducing glutathione and increasing oxidative stress[28]. Animal experiments were very promising in suggesting that aldose reductase inhibition could prevent the development of, but subsequent clinical trials with sorbinil[29], ponalrestat[30], and tolrestat[31] failed to demonstrate any slowdown of DR. However, these drugs may have been undertitrated and/or unable to reach the target tissues in effective concentrations, so that studies with other aldose reductase inhibitors that possess better bioavailability could still yield interesting results.

Advanced Glycation End Products Inhibitors

Chronically increased amounts of glucose amplify the physiological process of nonenzymatic protein glycosylation (glycation). Glucose forms labile links with the N-terminal and side-chain lysine radicals within proteins. Such links tend to turn into stable Amadori products, leading to degradation of both structural and functional proteins and accelerated aging. While most glycated proteins are eliminated in physiological conditions, they accumulate in if there is diabetes and undergo further structural arrangements with the formation of AGE[32], which, in turn, are implicated in the development of vascular lesions. Aminoguanidine, a compound that prevents AGE formation and that proved promising in the prevention of DR in animal models[33], was studied in a clinical trial but this was stopped in course due to safety considerations.

Antioxidants

The above pathways have so far been studied separately and every mechanism attacked with a specific compound. However, a unifying hypothesis was put forward recently, according to which oxidative stress might represent the common denominator of damage induced by hyperglycemia, through increased production of reactive oxygen species. These, in turn, would activate aldose reductase, induce DAG formation/PKC activation, increase AGE production, and activate the pleiotropic transcription nuclear factor κB[34-35]. Blocking all such pathways in a combined approach could obviously be extremely useful to prevent the progression of DR. Indeed, intracellular metabolism of excess glucose induces overproduction of superoxide, and inhibiting superoxide formation can reduce the production of sorbitol, AGE, and PKC activation. However, although, α-tocopherol prevented hemodynamic alterations in diabetic rats[36], AGE production occurs also through nonoxidative reactions, and a study of 387 patients with T2DM failed to demonstrate any protective effect for such antioxidants as vitamins C and E and β-carotene on retinal microvascular complication[37].

Thiamine and Benfotiamine

Blockade of the unifying mechanism of the pathogenesis of diabetic microangiopathy may be obtained through another, more radical, approach to the correction of the metabolic imbalances induced by high glucose/hyperglycemia. Thiamine (vitamin B1) is the cofactor of 3 enzymes involved in glycolysis and Kreb's cycle: transketolase, which shifts 2,3-diphosphoglycerate (2,3-DPG) into the pentose phosphate shunt, pyruvate dehydrogenase, which links pyruvate to acetyl-CoA and channels them into the Kreb's cycle, and α-ketoglutarate dehydrogenase, which accelerates the Kreb's cycle by turning α-ketoglutarate into succinyl-CoA. The net result is facilitation of glucose metabolism, which, in non-insulin-dependent complication-prone tissues, is critically busy in diabetes, with accumulation of highly reactive metabolites that, like 2,3-DPG, play a key role in the synthesis of AGE and the activation of DAG/PKC. In our laboratory, we were able to show that thiamine corrects increased lactate and AGE formation, along with reduced replication induced by high glucose in cultured endothelial cells[38]. These and other data were corroborated by the findings of Hammes et al. 2003, who reported that benfotiamine (a lipophilic analogue that can be administered orally) blocks the hexosamine pathway, AGE production, the PKC-DAG pathway, and nuclear factor κB up-regulation in both cell culture and experimental animals. More importantly, inhibition of these 3 major pathways of hyperglycemia-induced damage by benfotiamine and thiamine was found to prevent retinopathy[39] and nephropathy in animals with experimental diabetes. Before thiamine administration can be proposed for the prevention/treatment of diabetic microangiopathy, evidence should be provided that diabetes is a thiamine deficient state, at least relevant to the increased requirements induced by hyperglycemia. So far, only 1 report described reduced circulating thiamine in diabetic patients compared with healthy controls[40].

Diabetic Retinopathy and Hyperlipidemia

There is no strong evidence to consider dyslipidemia as a risk factor for macular edema or the progression of DR. The Hoorn study demonstrated an association between total and low-density lipoprotein cholesterol and the presence of retinal hard exudates[41]. Another study showed that aggressive lowering of blood lipids was followed by the disappearance of retinal hard exudates in 2 patients with diabetic macular disease. There is only anecdotal evidence on the role of statins in reducing the number of exudates, and a randomized trial could help clarify weather these drugs could be of any value in the treatment of exudative maculopathy, even in patients without dyslipidemia[42].

Anti-Angiogenic Agents

Diffuse retinal ischemia and hypoxia are presumably responsible for the release of angiogenic factors, such as VEGF, IGF I, and hepatocyte growth factor that represent powerful stimuli for neovascularization. VEGF is produced in the neuroretina and may play a pivotal role in the development of proliferative retinopathy. High levels of VEGF are found in the vitreous of patients undergoing vitrectomy in the presence of active retinal or iris neovascularization[43]. Blocking VEGF synthesis and vitreal injection of anti-VEGF antibodies prevented retinal neovascularization in animal models. Another attractive perspective is the blockade of the VEGF receptors 1 and 2, the expression of which is altered in the vascular endothelium of diabetic patients[44]. Pigment epithelium-derived factor (PEDF) is a potent intraocularly produced inhibitor of angiogenesis. The levels of VEGF are increased and those of PEDF decreased in PDR[45]. Abnormal production or secretion of VEGF and PEDF can induce retinal damage[46] and intraperitoneal administration of PEDF inhibits neovascularization in new born mice[47]. Recent studies further support an association between DR and increased VEGF concentrations in ocular fluids and suggest that treatment with thalidomide may be of benefit in streptozotocin-induced diabetic rats because thalidomide blocks the rise of VEGF. ACE inhibitors might also attenuate VEGF overexpression in PDR by inhibiting the local effects of angiotensin II[48].

Intravitreal anti-VEGF agents: VEGF has been identified as having a major role in the genesis of diabetic retinopathy, with increased levels in animals with experimental diabetes and in the vitreous of patients with diabetic retinopathy. Intravitreal VEGF administration in experimental animals duplicates many features of diabetic retinopathy. Thus, agents that attenuate VEGF action are very attractive because they are able to reduce permeability and neovascularization, the hallmarks of DME and PDR, respectively[49]. In general, systemically administered drugs reach the retinochoroidal tissue via blood circulation. However, because the BRB limits the influx of drugs into the retina, large amounts of the drug must be administered to maintain therapeutic concentrations. Regarding anti-VEGF agents, this would lead to systemic inhibition of angiogenesis, which could compromise critical vascular response to ischemic events in diabetic patients with cardiovascular, cerebrovascular, or peripheral vascular disease. Moreover, hypertension and proteinuria (two surrogate markers of systemic VEGF inhibition) as well as the impairment of wound healing are other potential consequences of blocking VEGF and would be particularly worrying to the diabetic population. By contrast, the local administration of anti-VEGF agents into the eye by means of intravitreal injections would avoid systemic adverse effects. However, this is invasive and a skilled specialist is required. In addition, in order to maintain effective levels, frequently repeated injections would be necessary, thus increasing local complications such as endophthalmitis, vitreous hemorrhage, retinal detachment, and traumatic cataract. Furthermore, although the eye is thought of as a closed and self-contained system, anti-VEGF drugs injected into the vitreous cavity pass into systemic circulation to varying degrees and could potentially cause the systemic adverse effects mentioned previously. At present four anti-VEGF agents are available: pegaptanib sodium (macugen; Pfizer), ranibizumab (lucentis; Genentech/Novartis), bevacizumab (avastin; Genentech), and aflibercept (Regeneron Pharmaceuticals/sanofi-aventis) and others are in phase trials (Table 4.2).

Table 4.2 Various anti VEGF drugs.

Agent	Company	Development stage	Development approach	Target	Route/ Frequency
Pegeptanib (Macugen)	OSI/ Eyetech	Marketed	Aptamer	VEGF165 isoform	ITV (every six weeks)
Bevacizumab (Avastin)	Genentech	Marketed	Monoclonal antibody	All VEGF A isoforms	IV or ITV (IV: every two weeks; ITV: to be determined)
Ranibizumab (Lucentis)	Genentech	Marketed	Monoclonal antibody fragment	All VEGF A isoforms	ITV (monthly)
Cand5	Acuity	Phase II	siRNA	VEGF-A mRNA	ITV (TBD)
Sima-027	SIRNA Allergen	Phase I/II	siRNA	VEGF-R1 mRNA	ITV (TBD)
AG-013958	Pfizer	Phase I/II	Tyrosine kinase inhibitor	VEGF-R2 and PEGFR	Sub tenon (TBD)
PTK787 (vatalanib)	Novartis	Phase I	Tyrosine kinase inhibitor	VEGF-R1, VEGF-R2, VEGF-R3	Oral (daily)
VEGF Trap	Regeneron	Phase I/II	Decoy receptor	All VEGF-A isoforms and PlGF	ITV (TBD)

Pegaptanib

It is a PEGylated (i.e., conjugated to polyethylene glycol) neutralizing RNA aptamer with an extremely high affinity for isoform 165 of VEGF ($VEGF_{165}$), which is the isoform that participates in pathological but not physiological neovascularization. Aptamers are modified nucleotides composed of single-stranded nucleic acids that adopt a specific three-dimensional conformation, allowing them to bind with high specificity and affinity to molecular targets in a manner similar to that of monoclonal antibodies. An important feature of aptamers is that they do not exhibit immunogenicity. Pegaptanib was approved by the U.S. Food and Drug Administration (FDA) for treatment of exudative (wet or neovascular) age-related macular disease (AMD) in December 2004[50].

Ranibizumab

Ranibizumab (trade name Lucentis®) is a recombinant humanized IgG1 kappa isotype monoclonal antibody fragment designed for intraocular use a full-length monoclonal antibody directed against VEGF. In contrast to pegaptanib, ranibizumab inhibits the biological activity of all isoforms of human VEGF and could be immunogenic. The FDA approved ranibizumab for wet AMD in June 2006. Ranibizumab binds to and inhibits the biologic activity of human vascular endothelial growth factor A. Ranibizumab has a molecular weight of approximately 48 kilodaltons and is produced by an E. coli expression system. Ranibizumab derived from the same parent murine antibody as bevacizumab. It is much smaller than the bevacizumab and has been affinity matured to provide stronger binding to VEGF-A. It is an anti-angiogenic that has been approved to treat the "wet" type of age-related macular degeneration (ARMD), a common form of age-related vision loss.

0.5 mg (0.05 mL) is recommended to be administered by intravitreal injection once a month (approximately 28 days). If monthly injections are not feasible, the regimen may be reduced to 1 injection every 3 months after the first 4 months[51].

Bevacizumab

Bevecizumab (trade name Avastin® is a recombinant humanized monoclonal IgG1 antibody that binds to and inhibits the biologic activity of human vascular endothelial growth factor (VEGF). Bevacizumab contains human framework regions and the complementarily-determining regions of a murine antibody that binds to VEGF. Bevacizumab is produced in a Chinese Hamster Ovary mammalian cell expression system has a molecular weight of approximately 149 kilodaltons[52]. 2.5 mg is recommended to be administered by intravitreal injection every two weeks. It was approved by the FDA in February 2004 for the treatment of disseminated colorectal cancer but not licensed for intraocular use. Nevertheless, intravitreal injection of bevacizumab has become a current off-label treatment by ophthalmologists for neovascular AMD because although it seems to be as effective as pegaptanib or ranimizumab, it is much cheaper.

VEGF Trap-Eye

VEGF Trap-Eye also known as flibercept and its ability to block all six VEGF proteins (VEGF-A to VEGF-E as well as placental growth factor), is a fusion protein comprised of segments of the extracellular domains of human VEGF receptors 1 (VEGFR1) and 2 (VEGFR2) fused to the constant region (Fc) of human IgG. Afilbercept is currently being used in clinical trials for both exudative AMD and DME[53]. A flibercept has a higher binding affinity than other anti-VEGF agents. This higher binding affinity translates into greater activity at lower biological levels and consequently, a longer duration of action. The results of prospective clinical trials using pegaptanib and ranibizumab in patients with AMD have been very impressive and have led to the design of specific trials for DME and PDR. At present, only a prospective double-blind multicenter dose-ranging controlled trial has been reported in diabetic patients. In this study 172 patients with DME were included, and the patients randomized to receive repeated intravitreal pegaptanib showed better visual outcomes, were more likely to show a reduction in retinal thickness and needed less additional focal laser ($P \geq 0.04$) at follow-up (36 weeks) than patients who received intravitreal sham injections. Retrospective data analysis of the eyes of 16 patients with PDR also showed regression of neovascularization. Uncontrolled studies using ranibizumab and bevacizumab have also found a rapid regression of retinal neovascularization, improvement of visual acuity and decrease of retinal thickness in DME, even in nonresponders to conventional treatment. However, the response to treatment of DME by VEGF blockade is not prolonged and is subject to significant variability. This is in distinct contrast to the rapid response of those with both iris and retinal neovascularization in PDR and of those with choroidal neovascularization in wet AMD. Interestingly, when the outcomes of intravitreal bevacizumab treatment of DME were compared with those of intravitreal cortisone (triamcinolone acetonide), better outcomes in terms of reduction of foveal thickness and visual results were found with triamcinolone. The extent to which VEGF blockade is beneficial for DME is currently being investigated in prospective clinical trials. Apart from their potential as isolated treatments for PDR and DME, intravitreal anti-VEGF agents, in particular bevacizumab, have been shown to be useful in increasing the short-term response to panretinal photocoagulation in high-risk PDR and also seem to be efficacious and safe as an adjuvant treatment to vitrectomy in severe PDR or vitreous hemorrhage. This is because intravitreal anti-VEGF agents reduce active neovascularization and vitreous hemorrhage, thus allowing a safe and efficient panretinal photocoagulation or pars plana vitrectomy to be performed while minimizing the risk of complications. Aflibercept has been recently tested in an exploratory study performed in five patients with DME. In this study, using a single intravitreal injection, Trap-Eye was well tolerated and preliminary evidence of bioactivity was detected. Taken together, these promising results present a new scenario in the management of diabetic retinopathy. Nevertheless, larger studies investigating not only the effectiveness but also the systemic adverse effects of these agents in the diabetic population are still needed. It is possible that a drug with more extensive and nonspecific anti-VEGF activity, such as pan-VEGF inhibitors (ranibizumab, bevacizumab, and aflibercept), could be more effective than a drug such as pegaptanib that selectively targets $VEGF_{165}$. In this regard, pegaptanib is substantially less effective than ranibizumab in AMD treatment. By contrast, given that $VEGF_{165}$ plays an essential role in pathological but not physiological neovascularization, pegaptanib could be the best option for avoiding systemic adverse effects in diabetic patients. In addition, long-term intravitreous injections of pan-VEGF inhibitors could lead to retinal neurodegeneration and an increased risk of circulation disturbances in the choriocapillaris. However, the theoretical advantage of selective blocking of VEGF165 by pegaptanib in terms of both systemic and local side effects remains to be demonstrated in head-to-head clinical trials.

SIRNA-027 (Sirna Therapeutics)

It is short interfering RNA (siRNA) that is designed to down regulate VEGF receptor-1, Sirna-027 reduces pathologic angiogenesis mediated by both VEGF and PIGF in experimental studies[54]. Sirna-027 is the first chemically optimized siRNA to be tested in a human clinical trial. At the time of manuscript preparation, the open-label, dose-escalation phase I study was ongoing for the treatment of wet AMD.

Tyrosine Kinase Inhibitors

Small molecule receptor tyrosine kinse inhibitors that target all VEGF receptors are being developed. For instance, vatalanib (PKT787), is a potent inhibitor of all known VEGF receptor tyrosine kinases (VEGFR1, VEGFR2 and VEGFR3), with a slightly greater potency against VEGFR1 and VEGFR2. Preclinical studies suggest that PKT787 induces dose dependent inhibition of VEGF-induced angiogenesis in growth factor implant models as well as tumor cell-driven angiogenesis models. In an animal model of retinal neovascularization, daily subcutaneous injections of PTK787 (10mg/kg) in neonatal mice significantly inhibited retinal vasculaization and a single ITV injection of PTK787 (40 µmol/l dose) reduced angioproliferative changes using the same murine model of oxygen-induced retinal neovascularization. Daily oral administration of PTK787 (25mg/kg) completely inhibited the neovascularization that develops in the subretinal space of rhodopsin/VEGF transgenic mice and daily oral administration (50mg/kg) for 14 consecutive days decreased choroidal neovascularization by approximately 80% in a laser induced model of choroidal neovascularization. Vatalanib is in clinical development as an antiangiogenic therapy for patients with cancer, and with oral administration of vatalanib once daily in a phase I study in combination with verteporfin photodynamic therapy in patients with neovascular AMD[55].

AG-013736

It is another small molecule receptor tyrosine kinase inhibitor that targets VEGF/platelet-derived growth factor receptor tyrosine kinases and has shown promise in a Phase II metastatic renal cell carcinoma study; however; it is not under clinical investigation in patients with neovascular AMD. A preclinical study of another small molecule receptor tyrosine kinase inhibitor, AG-013736 which is a selective inhibitor of VEGFR and PDGFR, found that it inhibited vascular development and induced capillary regression in rats. Preclinical studies in cynomolgus monkeys that received sub tenon administration of AG-013736 found effective choroidal concentrations and minimal systemic exposure of AG-013736. Similiarly preclinical trials results from 21 patients with subfoveal CNV secondary to AMD who received AG-013736 is associated with minimal systemic exposure and mild adverse events. A phase I/II, randomized, masked, dose-escalation study of AG-013736 is under way in patients with subfoveal CNV secondary to AMD. **Table 4.3** shows the biochemical changes and various drugs available for the treatment of diabetic retinopathy.

Table 4.3 Various drugs available for the treatment of diabetic retinopathy.

Increase activity	Mechanism	Drugs/Treatment	Effective	Dosages form	Dose
Vascular endothelial growth factor (VEGF)	VEGF is the substance directly responsible for simulating vasoproliferation and increased perme-ability. PKC is a signal transducer switch to activate or inhibit the activity of VEGF and VEGF inturn activate PKC and cause fluid leakage, cell proliferation and inflammation.	Bevacizumab (Avastin, Genentech, Inc., South San Francisco,CA) Ranibizumab (Lucentis, Genentech, Inc.) Pegaptanib (Macugen, OSI/Eyetech, Melville, NY) VEGF Trap-eye (Regeneron Pharmaceuticals, Inc.,)	DME and PDR	Intravitreal Injection	Bevacizumab (1.25 mg and high as 2.5 mg),. Ranibizumab (0.5 mg) [19]. Pegaptanib (0.3mg), and VEGF trap (0.5 mg).
Inflammation (Steroids)	Diabetes leads to maladaptive chronic inflammatory response in retinal endothelial and neural cells, resulting in VEGF production and recruitment of inflammatory mediators, causing increased vascular permeability, capillary non-perfusion, neurodegeneration, and neovascularization. Steroids reduce inflammation, fluid leakage and close the tight junctions between endothelial cells.	Triamcinolone acetonide, Triamcinolone acetonide implant (I-vation), Flucinolone acetonide implant (Retisert), Dexamethasone implant (Posidurex). Corticosteroids	Short term benefits but in the long term, needs repeated application of intravitreal injection due to recurrence of DME.	Intravitreal Injection	Triamcinolone acetonide (1-8 mg, common dose 4 mg).

Table 4.3 Contd...

48

Increase activity	Mechanism	Drugs/Treatment	Effective	Dosages form	Dose
Renin-angiotensin system (RAAS)	Intraocular remin-angiotensin system gets up-regulated in diabetes and stimulates VEGF expression in retinal vascular endothelial cells. RAAS inhibitors reduce blood pressure, ameliorating the hydrostatic process that exacerbates fluid leakage.	ACE inhibitors: lisinopril enalapril, ramipril, candesartan, losartan and spironolactone.	PDR	Intravitreal Injection	Enalapril (10 mg/day).
Enzymes	The vitreous in diabetic patients undergoes structural changes leading to collagen cross-linking and vitreomacular traction worsening the DME. Newly formed vessels use the posterior hyaloid face as a scaffold to grow. The retracting vitreous pulls on these vessels and is responsible for both vitreous hemorrhage and retinal detachment in PDR.	Hyaluronidase, Plasmin, Microplasmin	PDR and DME	Intravitreal, Phase III trial	Hyaluronidase (5 U) alone is ineffective, whereas plasmin (0.25 U) alone induces partial PVD, a very dangerous state for the diabetic eye. Combination of hyaluronidase and plasmin can induce complete PVD in 12-week old diabetic rats.

Table 4.3 *Contd...*

Increase activity	Mechanism	Drugs/Treatment	Effective	Dosages form	Dose
Carbonic anhydrase	Extracellular carbonic anhydrase increases retinal vascular permeability by increasing pH, leading to kallikrein-mediated proteolytic activation of kinin.	Acetazolamide	DME and PDR	Oral	Acetazolamide.
Oxidative stress	Hyperglycaemia increases production of reactive-oxygen species (free radicals), leading to activation of protein kinase C, formation of advanced glycation end-products (AGE), activation of the polyol pathway, and VEGF production. The antioxidants suppress production of the growth factor VEGF, which promotes abnormal blood vessels in the retina.	Vitamin C, Viamin E and Benfotiamine.	DME and PDR	Intravitreal injection	Benfotiamine, a lipid soluble derivative of water soluble vitamin B1 (thiamine), has been used for the past 12 years in Europe for the treatment of neuropathy, retinopathy as well as heart and circulatory conditions and has shown no adverse effects.
Growth hormone and insulin growth factor (IGF)	Growth hormone and IGF modulate the function of retinal endothelial precursor cells and drive retinal angiogenesis in response to hypoxia; IGF-1 can also disrupt the blood-retina barrier and increase retinal vascular permeability.	Growth harmone inhibitors like- Octreotide	DME and PDR	Intravitreal Injection	Octreotide 10-30 mg per 5 mL.

Table 4.3 *Contd...*

Increase activity	Mechanism	Drugs/Treatment	Effective	Dosages form	Dose
Sorbitol	Hyperglycaemia increases glucose flux through the polyol pathway, via which aldose reductase converts glucose into intracellular sorbitol, possibly inducing osmotic damage to retinal endothelial cells and pericytes.	Aldose rectase inhibitors like-Ranirestat, Epalrestat	DME	Oral	Ranirestat (40 and 80 mg for neuropath). Epalrestat administration lowers Nepsilon (carboxymethyl) lysine (CML).
AGE	Hyperglycaemia induces non-enzymatic glycation of proteins to form AGE, possibly contributing to retinal perictye loss, microaneurysm formation, and vascular endothelial damage	Pimagedine reduces Progression of Retinopathy and Lowers Lipid Levels in Patients with Type 1 Diabetes Mellitus	PDR	Oral	Pimagedine 300 mg or 600 mg BID.
Peroxisome proliferator-activated receptor gamma (PPAR-γ) agonists	Due to uncontrolled of diabetes hyperglycemic takes place which increase the activity of VEGF and neovascularization takes place.	PPARγ agonist rosiglitazone maleate, Rosiglitazone maleate	retinal leukostasis and retinal leakaged and Recently, Shen et al. (2008) PDR	Oral	Rosiglitazone 2 mg twice a day or 4 mg/day.
Protein kinase C	Hyperglycaemia increases activation of retinal cellular protein-kinase C, leading to increased vasoactive mediators, with adverse structural and functional retinal vascular changes.	Midostaurin, Ruboxistaurin, Rottlein, Indolocarbazoles, Bisindoylmaleimides	DME and PDR	Ruboxistaurin (Oral)	Ruboxistaurin (32 mg per day, Phase III trial).

Limitations of Ranibizumab/Bevacizumab and their Intravitreal Formulation

Since these drugs are high molecular weight and protenious in nature, there are various issues related to their stability and permeability through ocular barriers like tear fluid-eye barrier, cornea, conjunctiva and blood ocular barriers. Moreover, they are available in the form of intravitreal injection (IVT) which itself have various usage limitations like elevation in intraocular pressure from baseline up to 25mm Hg which leads to iridocyclitis, endopthalmitis and ischemic central retinal vein occlusion. Other ocular adverse events occurring is > 10% of ranibizumab treated patients were conjunctival hemorrhage, iridocyclitis, iritis, retinal hemorrhage, retinal detachment, traumatic cataract and reduction in visual acuity. Ranibizumab has course duration of 24 months, this suggests that the cost of treatment may exceed $ 58,488.00 and the delivery of IVT should be carried out by a licensed and qualified physician under controlled aseptic technique through a 5-micron 19-gauge filter attached to a 1-cc tuberculin syringe. The filter needle is replaced with a sterile 30-gauge x 1/2-inch needle for the intravitreal injection. 0.05 ml is injected into the eye under aseptic conditions using sterile gloves, a sterile drape and a sterile eyelid speculum. The eye is ordinarily prepared with Betadyne and adequate anesthesia. Each vial is used for only one eye. All these procedures lead to patient non-compliance. There are various approaches to overcome these limitations by:

1. **Increasing the absorption** through the application of physical methods (iontophoresis/ phonophoresis), co-administration with permeation enhancers (BL-9, Brij 78, Brij 99, Fusidic acid, Saponin), incorporation into liposomes, niosomes, or other carriers.

2. **Minimizing metabolism** through covalent attachment to a polymer, chemical modification of primary structure, targeting to specific tissues and co-administration with enzyme inhibitor.

3. **Prolonging drug levels** through use of bioadhesives, liposomes, niosomes, proniosomes, polymeric nanoparticulate systems, solid-lipid nanoparticulated system or other carrier systems.

Ruboxistaurin (LY333531)

LY333531 (32mg OD for 1 month, under phase III trial) is a highly selective potent reversible PKC β inhibitor. LY333531 is present in the form of seven salts namely hydrochloride, sulphate, mesylate, succinate, tartrate, acetate and phosphate. 43% of FDA approved marketed salts are hydrochloride and only 2% have been marketed as mesylate salts. Apart from mesylate salt rest were eliminated either due to poor crystallinity, low solubility and impurity issues. The AUC 3.89 and C_{max} 896 $\pm$ 243ng/mL of mesylate salt is higher than its hydrochloride salt i.e 1.62 and 400 $\pm$ 142ng/ml. The metabolite of LY333531 is N-desmethyl Ruboxistaurin (LY338522) was found to be equally active with C_{max} value of 2455 $\pm$ 930ng/ml [35, 36]. LY333531 is highly selective inhibitor with an IC_{50} value 5.9nm and 4.7nm for PKC βII and βI respectively but PKC isoforms namely α, γ, δ, ϵ and η get inhibited by an IC_{50} values 360nm, 300nm, 250nm, 600nm and 52nm respectively[56-57].

Expected Problems Associated with Oral Targeting

PKC is a signal transducer which activates or inhibits VEGF and VEGF in turn activates or inhibit PKC. Therefore, PKC and VEGF form a vicious cycle in an intracellular process of biochemical pathophysiology of neovascularization. Since PKC family is widely distributed through out the body and the inhibition of PKC isoforms would also suppress VEGF therefore, oral dosage form of Ruboxistaurin is likely to have serious, perhaps fatal and systemic consequences[58] like increased risk of stroke and impared reparative neurogenesis in brain, impairment of collateral vessels development in heart, vasculature hypertension, collapse of capillary loops, impaired podocyte function and protein urea in kidney, neuropathy and impaired motor sensation in peripheral nervous system and impairment of wound healing. Comparatively, since PKC β is present at high level in retina, ocular targeting of Ruboxistaurin using novel formulation approaches will be more beneficial in the treatment of diabetic retinopathy with out any systemic and peripheral side effects.

Herbal Products with Anti-Angiogenic Activity

Angiogenic modulators are present in a wide range of plant products, some of which are also consumed on a daily basis through diets. Herbal products derived from specific medicinal plants known for their curative properties on chronic angiogenesis-dependent conditions are also gaining recognition for their principal active agents.

Curcuma Longa (Turmeric)

The staple in India's armoury of wound-healing plants is the common spice plant C. longa, used for injuries, burns, and an all-purpose, topical anti-inflammatory[59]. The principal active substance is curcumin. The use of curcumin as an inhibitor of angiogenesis has only recently been appreciated, despite great interest in this natural product for cancer chemoprevention. The local delivery of curcuminoid pellets (2 mg), implanted in the cornea of rabbits, blocked angiogenesis induced by fibroblast growth factor 2 and even oral delivery of curcuminoid to mice blocked angiogenesis induced by the same growth factor in the mouse corneal model of neovascularization[60]. The mechanism of curcumin is believed to be dependent on disease contexts. The one of curcumin's target is kinase that is responsible for activating the multipurpose signaling complex, acting as a central modulator of stress response. The COP9 signalosome activates the expression of VEGF in tumour cells providing the cells with survival advantage by stimulating blood vessels. Curcumin's anti-angiogenic activity causes the inhibition of VEGF expression.

Panax Ginseng (Ginseng)

The root of P. ginseng is highly reversed in the Far East for their medical properties[61]. The main active principles that target blood vessels are ginsenosides. Unlike turmeric, whose dual actions of angiomodulatory activity can be shown to result from curcumin, the activity of ginseng is attributed to different subclasses of ginsenosides such as Rb_1 and Rg_1. At doses of 1 nmol/L to 1 μmol/L, 20(R)-Rg_3, showed dose-dependent inhibition of endothelial cell proliferation and inhibition of VEGF-induced chemoinvasion and tube formation. Rg_3 also reduces the expression of MMP-2 and MMP-9, metalloproteinnases that are involved in tube formation and invasion. Like Rg_3, the ginsenoside Rb_1 also demonstrates anti-angiogenic activity. When Rb1 is combined with Rg_1, in different amounts of ginsenosides can either induce or restrict blood vessel growth based on their compositional ratios. This is because of panaxatriols represented by Rg_1 and Rb_1 have proangiogenic activity. The proangiogenic mechanism of Rg_1, which induces endothelial cell proliferation, is related to stimulation genes involved in cytoskeleton dynamics, cell-cell adhesion and migration.

Withania Somniferia (Ashwagandha)

The herb plant has invigorating and tonic uses in Ayurvedic medicine[62]. Some of the popular uses of the roots of this plant are for the treatment of arthritic conditions and for bleeding disorders that result from menstrual dysfunction. Hypothesising that an underlaying angiogenic mechanism is targeted by the extract of W. somnifera, investigated the extracts of this plant for the presence of angiogenesis inhibitors by exploiting the 3D-ECSA. The combination of bioactivity testing in the 3D-ECSA along with assessment in the Matrigel model of angiogenesis revealed that the angiogenesis inhibitory activity present in the methanolic extracts was enriched about fivefold upon further fractionation into chloroform-soluble substances. In assessing the molecular mechanism targeted by the chloroform-enriched fraction, it was found that the DNA binding activity of transcription factor NF-κB was specifically and potential inhibited by the chloroform extract (IC_{50} 10μg/mL).

Hypericum Perforatum (St John's Wort)

It is widely used herb for depression, is also the source of anti-angiogenic agents, hypericin and hyperforin. Angiogenesis inhibitory activity of hyperforin has attracted attention not only to the border uses of this plant in human disease, but also to the potential side effects[63], specially so in patients who may have other vascular complications where an anti-angiogenic agent would have contradiction. The mode of action of hyperforin is due to inhibition of MMP-9 expression, an enzyme that is responsible for basement membrane degradation during blood vessel growth. In addition, hyperforin inhibits microtubules which prevent endothelial cells forming capillary tubes. In other models hyperforin was shown to target components within G-protein signaling cascade that regulate Ca^{2+} homeostasis and inhibit neutrophil invasion and block inflammatory activation, suggesting that the target of this natural product is present on both vascular and inflammatory components that act in synergy during many angiogenic diseases. A dose of Hypericum extract 900 mg/day used as an antidepressant (which supplies 0.4 μmol/L of hyperforin) was shown to down-regulate production of angiogenic cytokine interferon-gamma in activated T-cell with concomitant inhibition of MMP-9 expression. On the other hand, hypericin is also a potent angiogenesis inhibitor that targets activity of a related proteinase, MT1-MMP and is also responsible for inhibiting signaling events that trigger MAP kinase. Hypericin administered at 2 mg/Kg intraperiteoneally, blocks activating phosphorylation of ERK1/2, which is required for the transactivation of hypoxia-inducible factor 1 alpha (HIF-1α) and in VEGF-induced blood vessel growth in models employing photodynamic therapy.

Camellia Sinensis (Green Tea)

Epidermiologesical evidences has raised the intrest in green tea consumption for prevention of cancers and cardiovascular diseases and research to identify the biologically active substances of tea extracts. One of the major ingredients of green tea, (-)epigallocatechin gallate (EGCG), a flavonoid, was shown to inhibit angiogenesis and have chemopreventive activity. Using data derived from rodent studies (Fassina et al, 2004), a phase 1 study of green tea extract was performed. A dose for antiangiogenic activity in humans was calculated to be $1g/m^2$ three times per day[64].

Vitis Vinifera (Red Grapes)

Red wine consumption is belived to be protective of the cardiovascular system, as evidenced in the prevention of the progression of atherosclerosis even in people who consume high amounts of red meat and cholesterol-containing foods[65]. This was thought to be due to the major cardioprotective polyphenolic compounds found in skins and seeds of red grapes. One of these red wine polyphenolic compounds (RWPC) is the natural product resveratrol. The antiangiogenic mechanisms of resveratrol are known to be complex; since it inhibits proliferation of endothelial cells at 25 µmol/L with inhibitory effects on cell migration and vessel tube formation occurring at 25-50 µmol/L. The inhibitory activity of resveratrol on metalloproteinases MMP-9 was observed at 6.25 µmol/L, whereas on MMP-2 activity was at 25 µmol/L. Reveratrol inhibits VEGF-induced angiogenesis by interfering with reactive oxygen species dependent Src kinase activation and down-regulates the expression of angiogenic cytokines, including interleukin-8 and VEGF. RWPCs show dose-dependent opposite effect on angiogenesis. In rats, 0.2 mg/Kg/day of RWPCs caused a pro-angiogenic effect while higher daily doses of 2 mg/kg of RWPC (equivalents found in seven glasses of red wine) showed anti-angiogenic activity in the post-ischaemic model of hind limb neovascularization. It was found that the low dose (1/10 glass) angiogenic effect occurs through overexpression of P13 kinase-AKT-NOS pathway leading to increased VEGF production without affecting MMP production.

Betulinic Acid

Betulinic acid (3β, hydroxy-lup-20(29)-en-28-oic acid) is a pentacyclic triterpenoid of plant origin that is widely distributed in the plant kingdom throughout the world. For example, considerable amounts of betulinic acid are available in the outer bark of a variety of tree species, e.g. white-barked birch trees. The reduced congener of betulinic acid, betulin (3β-lup-20(29)-en-3,28-diol), was one of the first natural products identified and isolated from plants in 1788. Betulinic acid exerts a number of biological activities. For example, betulinic acid has been shown to have antitumor properties. To this end, it is interesting to note that white birch bark (Betula alba) which contains betulinic acid, has been used by Native Americans as a folk remedy. Betulinic acid has also been reported to inhibit aminopeptidase N, an enzyme that is involved in the regulation of angiogenesis and overexpressed in several cancers. In addition, betulinic acid was reported to exert antiangiogenic effects by inhibiting growth factor-induced *in vitro* angiogenesis in endothelial cells, possibly by affecting mitochondrial functions. Further, the antiangiogenic activity of betulinic acid was attributed to activation of selective proteasome-dependent degradation of the transcription factors specificity protein 1 (Sp1), Sp3, and Sp4, which regulate vascular endothelial growth (VEGF) expression. Compared to betulinic acid, 20,29-dihydro-betulinic acid derivatives were claimed to posses better anti-angiogenic properties as betulinic acid. Also, betulinic acid was shown to inhibit the catalytic activity of topoisomerase I. Furthermore, betulinic acid exerts context-dependant effects on the cell cycle. While betulinic acid was found to reduce expression of p21 protein in melanoma cells, an increase of p21 protein was observed upon treatment with betulinic acid in glioblastoma cells. Alterations in cell cycle progression in response to betulinic acid were also highly dependant on individual cell lines. Whether betulinic acid-mediated cell cycle changes are linked to its antitumor activity remains to be addressed in future studies[66].

References

1. Ferris III FL, Davis MD, Aiello LM, Treatment of diabetic retinopathy, N Engl J Med, 1999, 341, 667– 678.

2. Drexler W, Morgner U, Ghanta R K, Karter FX, Shuman JS, Fujimoto JG, Ultra-high-resolution ophthalmic optical coherence tomography, Nat Med, 2001, 7, 502– 507.

3. Rutledge BK, Wallow IH, Poulsen GL, Sub-pigment epithelial membranes after photocoagulation for diabetic macular edema, Arch Ophthalmol, 1993, 111, 608-613.

4. The Diabetes Control and Complications Trial (DCCT) Research Group, The effect of intensive treatment of diabetes on the development and progression of long-term complications in insulin-dependent diabetes mellitus, N Engl J Med, 1993, 329, 977– 986.

5. UKPDS Group, Intensive blood-glucose control with sulphonylureas or insulin compared with conventional treatment and risk of complications in patients with type 2 diabetes (UKPDS 33), Lancet, 1998a, 352, 837– 853.

6. The Diabetes Control and Complications Trial (DCCT) Research Group, The effect of intensive diabetes treatment on the progression of diabetic retinopathy in insulin-dependent diabetes mellitus, Arch Ophthalmol, 1995, 113, 36– 51.

7. Writing Team for the Diabetes Control and Complications Trial/Epidemiology of Diabetes Interventions and Complications Research Group, Effect of intensive therapy on the microvascular complications of type 1 diabetes mellitus, JAMA, 2002, 287, 2563– 2569.

8. Atherton A, Hill DW, Keen H, Young S, Edwards EJ, The effect of acute hyperglycaemia on the retinal circulation of the normal cat, Diabetologia, 1980, 18, 233– 237.

9. Grunwald JE, Riva CE, Petrig BL, Strict control of glycaemia: effects on blood flow in the large retinal vessels and in the macular microcirculation, Br J Ophthalmol, 1995, 79, 735– 741.

10. Chantelau E and Kohner EM, Why some cases of retinopathy worsen when diabetic control improves, Br Med J, 1997, 315, 1105– 1106.

11. Poulaki V, Qin W, Joussen AM, Hurlbut P, Wiegand SJ, Rudge J, Yancopoulos GD, Adamis AP, Acute intensive insulin therapy exacerbates diabetic blood retinal barrier breakdown via hypoxia-inducible factor 1-alpha and VEGF, J Clin Invest, 2002, 109, 805– 815.

12. Klein R, Klein BE, Lee KE, Cruickshanks KJ, Moss SE, The incidence of hypertension in insulin-dependent diabetes, Arch Intern Med, 1996, 156, 622– 627.

13. Suzuma I, Hata Y, Clermont A, Pokras F, Rook SL, Suzuma K, Feener EP, Aiello LP, Cyclic stretch and hypertension induced retinal VEGF-R2 (KDR) expression: potential mechanisms for exacerbation of diabetic retinopathy by hypertension, Diabetes, 2001, 50, 444– 454.

14. Rassam SM, Patel V, Kohner EM, The effect of experimental hypertension on retinal vascular autoregulation in humans: a mechanism for the progression of diabetic retinopathy, Exp Physiol, 1995, 80, 53–68.

15. Harper R, Ennis CN, Heaney AP, Sheridan B, Gormley M, Atkinson AB, Johnston GD, Bell PM, A comparison of the effects of low and conventional dose thiazide diuretic on insulin action in hypertensive patients with NIDDM, Diabetologia, 1995, 38, 853– 859.

16. The Blood Pressure Lowering Treatment Trialists' Collaboration, Effects of ACE inhibitors, calcium antagonist, and other bloodpressure- lowering drugs: results of prospectively designed overviews of randomized trials, Lancet, 2000, 356, 1955– 1964.

17. Wakisaka M, Yoshinari M, Nakamura S, Asano T, Sonoki K, Shi A, Takata Y, Fujishima M, Suppression of sodium-dependent glucose uptake by captopril improves high-glucose induced morphological and functional changes of cultured bovine retinal pericytes, Microvasc Res, 1999, 58, 215–223.

18. Zhang JZ, Gao L, Widness M, Xi X, Kem TS, Captopril inhibits glucose accumulation in retinal cells in diabetes, Invest Ophthalmol Vis Sci, 2003, 44, 40001– 40005.

19. Nagisa Y, Shintani A, Nakagawa S, The angiotensin II receptor antagonist candesartan cilexetil (TCV-116) ameliorates retinal disorders in rats, Diabetologia, 2001 44, 883–888.

20. Chaturvedi N, Sjolie AK, Stephenson JM, Abrahamian H, Castellarin A, Rogulia-Pepeonik Z, Fuller JH, Effect of lisinopril on progression of retinopathy in normotensive people with type 1 diabetes, Lancet, 1998, 35, 28– 31.

21. Chaturvedi N, Sjoelie AK, Svensson A, The Diabetic Retinopathy Candesartan Trials (DIRECT) Programme, rationale and study design, J Renin Angiotensin Aldosterone Syst, 2002, 3, 255– 261.

22. Colwell JA, Halushka PV, Sarji K, Levine J, Sagel J, Nair RM, Altered platelet function in diabetes mellitus, Diabetes, 1976, 25, 826– 831.

23. Joussen AM, Poulaki V, Mitsiades N, Kirchhof B, Koizumi K, Dohmen S, Adamis AP, Nonsteroidal anti-inflammatory drugs prevent early diabetic retinopathy via TNF-suppression, FASEB J, 2002, 16, 438– 440.

24. Khan ZA, and Chakrabarti S, Growth factors in proliferative diabetic retinopathy, Exp Diabesity Res, 2003, 4, 287– 301.

25. Simo R, Lecube A, Sararols L, Garcia-Arumi J, Segura RM, Casamitjana R, Hernandez C, Deficit of somatostatin-like immunoreactivity in the vitreous fluid of diabetic patient's possible role in the development of proliferative diabetic retinopathy, Diabetes Care, 2002, 25, 2282– 2286.

26. Koya D and King GL, Protein kinase C activation and the development of diabetic complications, Diabetes, 1998, 47, 859– 866.

27. Aiello LP, Davis MD, Milton RC, Sheetz J, Arora V, Vignati L, Initial results of the protein kinase C beta inhibitor Diabetic Macular Edema Study (PKC-DMES), Diabetologia, 2003, 46, A42.

28. Giugliano D, Ceriello A, Paolisso G, Oxidative stress and diabetic vascular complications, Diabetes Care, 1996, 19, 257– 267.

29. Sorbinil Retinopathy Trial Research Group, A randomized trail of sorbinil, an aldose reductase inhibitor, in diabetic retinopathy, Doc Ophthalmol, 1991, 78, 153– 159.

30. Arauz-Pacheco C, Ramirez LC, Pruneda L, Sanborn GE, Rosenstock J, Raskin P, The effect of the aldose reductase inhibitor, ponalrestat, on the progression of diabetic retinopathy, J Diabetes Complications, 1992, 6, 131–137.

31. Van Gerven JM, Boot JP, Lemkes HH, Van Best JA, Effects of aldose reductase inhibition with tolrestat on diabetic retinopathy in a six months double blind trial, Doc Ophthalmol, 1994, 87, 335– 365.

32. Singh R, Barden A, Mori T, Beilin L, Advanced glycation end-products: a review, Diabetologia, 2001, 44, 129–146.

33. Mizutani M, Gerhardinger C, Lorenzi M, Muller cell changes in human diabetic retinopathy, Diabetes, 1998, 47, 815– 820.

34. Nishikawa T, Edelstein D, Brawnlee M, The missing link: a single unifying mechanism for diabetic complications, Kidney Int Suppl, 2000, 58, S26–S30.

35. Nishikawa T, Edelstein D, Du XL, Yamagishi S, Matsumura T, Kaneda Y, Yorek MA, Neebe D, Oates PJ, Hamnes HP, Giardino I, Brownlee M, Normalizing mitochondrial superoxide production blocks three pathways of hyperglycaemic damage, Nature, 2000, 404, 87–790.

36. Kunisaki M, Bursell SE, Clermont AC, Ishii H, Ballas LM, Jirousek MR, Umeda F, Nawata H, King GL, Vitamin E prevents diabetes-induced abnormal retinal blood flow via the diacylglycerol-protein kinase C pathway, Am J Physiol, 1995, 269, E239– E246.

37. Mayer-Davis EJ, Bell RA, Reboussin BA, Rushing J, Marshall JA, Hamman RF, Antioxidant nutrient intake and diabetic retinopathy: the San Louis Valley diabetes study, Ophthalmology, 1998, 105, 2264– 2270.

38. La Selva M, Beltramo E, Pagnozzi F, Bena E, Molinatti PA, Molinatti GM, Porta M, Thiamine corrects delayed replication and decreases production of lactate and advanced glycation end-products in bovine retinal and human umbilical vein endothelial cells cultured under high glucose conditions, Diabetologia, 1996, 39, 1263– 1268.

39. Hammes HP, Du X, Edelstein D, Taguchi T, Matsumura T, Ju Q, Lin J, Bierhaus A, Nawroth P, Hannak D, Neumaier M, Bergfeld R, Giardino I, Brownlee M, Benfotiamine blocks three major pathways of hyperglycemic damage and prevents experimental diabetic retinopathy, Nat Med, 2003, 9, 294– 299.

40. Saito N, Kimura M, Kuchiba A, Itokawa Y, The relationship between blood thiamine levels and dietary thiamine content in diabetic outpatients and healthy subjects, J Nutr Sci Vitaminol, 1987, 33, 431–438.

41. Van Leiden HA, Dekker JM, Moll AC, Nijpels G, Heine RJ, Bouter LM, Stehouwer CD, Polak BC, Blood pressure, lipids, and obesity are associated with retinopathy: the Hoorn study, Diabetes Care, 2002, 25, 1320–1325.

42. Chowdhury TA, Hopkins D, Dodson PM, Valfidis GC, The role of serum lipids in exudative diabetic maculopathy: is there a place for lipid lowering therapy? Eye, 2002, 16, 689– 693.

43. Blaauwgeers HG, Holtkamp GM, Rutten H, Witmer AN, Koolwijk P, Partanen TA, Alitalo K, Kroon ME, Kijlstra A, Van Hinsbergh VW, Schlingemann RO, Polarized vascular endothelial growth factor secretion by human retinal pigment epithelium and localization of vascular endothelial growth factor receptors on the inner choriocapillaris: evidence for a trophic paracrine relation, Am J Pathol, 1999, 155, 421–428.

44. Adamis AP, Shima DT, Tolentino MJ, Gragoudas ES, Ferrara N, Folkman J, D'Amore PA, Miller JW, Inhibition of vascular endothelial growth factor prevents retinal ischemia-associated iris neovascularization in a nonhuman primate, Arch Ophthalmol, 1996, 114, 66–71.

45. Stellmach V, Crawford SE, Zhou W, Bouck N, Prevention of ischemia-induced retinopathy by the natural ocular antiangiogenic agent pigment epithelium-derived factor, Proc Natl Acad Sci USA, 2001, 98, 2593– 2597.

46. Gao G, Li Y, Zhang D, Gee S, Crosson C, Unbalanced expression of VEGF and PEDF in ischemia-induced retinal neovascularization, FEBS Lett, 2001, 489, 270– 276.

47. Witmer AN, Blaauwgeers HG, Weich HA, Alitalo K, Vrensen GF, Schlingemann RO, Altered expression patterns of VEGF receptors in human diabetic retina and in experimental VEGF-induced retinopathy in monkey, Invest Ophthalmol Vis Sci, 2002, 43, 849–857.

48. Hogeboom van Buggenum IM, Polak BC, Reichert-Thoen JW, de Vries-Knoppert WA, Van Hinsbergh VW, Tangelder GJ, Angiotensin converting enzyme inhibiting therapy is associated with lower vitreous vascular endothelial growth factor concentrations in patients with proliferative diabetic retinopathy, Diabetologia, 2002, 45, 203– 209.

49. Bhagat N, Grigorian RA, Tutela A, Diabetic macular edema: pathogenesis and treatment, Surv Ophthalmol, 2009, 54, 1–32.

50. Cunningham Jr ET, Adamis AP, Altaweel M, Aiello LP, Bressler NM, D'Amico DJ, Goldbaum M, Guyer DR, Katz B, Patel M, Schwartz SD, Macugen Diabetic Retinopathy Study Group, A phase II randomized double-masked trial of pegaptanib, an anti-vascular endothelial growth factor aptamer, for diabetic macular edema, Ophthalmology, 2005, 112, 1747–1757.

51. Chun DW, Heier JS, Topping TM, Duker JS, Bankert JM, A pilot study of multiple intravitreal injections of ranibizumab in patients with center-involving clinically significant diabetic macular edema, Ophthalmology, 2006, 113, 1706–1712.

52. Arevalo JF, Wu L, Sanchez JG, Maia M, Saravia MJ, Fernandez CF, Evans T, Intravitreal bevacizumab (Avastin) for proliferative diabetic retinopathy: 6-months followup, Eye, 2009b, 23, 117–123.

53. Do DV, Nguyen QD, Shah SM, Browning DJ, Haller JA, Chu K, Yang K, Cedarbaum JM, Vitti RL, Ingerman A, Campochiaro PA, An exploratory study of the safety, tolerability and bioactivity of a single intravitreal injection of vascular endothelial growth factor Trap-Eye in patients with diabetic macular oedema, Br J Ophthalmol, 2009, 93, 144–149.

54. Reich SJ, Fosnot J, Kuroki A, small interferring RNA (si RNA) targeting VEGF effectively inhibits ocular neovasculrization in a mouse model, Mol Vis, 2003, 9, 210-216.

55. Maier P, Unsoeld AS, Junker B, Intravitreal injection of specific receptor tyrosine kinase inhibitor PTK787/ZK222584 improves ischaemia-induced retinopathy in a rat, Graefe's Arch clin Exp Ophthalmol, 2005, 243, 593-600.

56. Ishii H, Koya D, King GL, Protein kinase C activation and its role in the development of vascular complications in diabetes mellitus, J Mol Med, 1998, 76, 21-31.

57. Way KJ, Chou E, King GL, Identification of PKC-isoformspecific biological actions using pharmacological approaches, Trends Pharmacol Sci, 2000, 21, 181-187.

58. Frank RN, Potential new medical therapies for diabetic retinopathy: Protein kinase C inhibitors, A J Ophthalmol, 2002, 133, 693-698.

59. Singh S. From exotic spice to modern drug? Cell, 2007, 130, 765-768.

60. Mohan R, Sivak J, Ashton P, Curcuminoids inhibit the angiogenic response stimulated by fibroblast growth factor-2, including expression of matrix metalloproteinase gelatinase B, J Biol Chem 2000, 275, 10405-10412.

61. Yue PY, Mak NK, Cheng YK, Pharmacogenomics and the Yin/Yang actions of ginseng: antitumor, angiomodulating and steroid-like activities of ginsenoside, Chin Med, 2007, 2, 6.

62. Begum VH and Sadique J, Long term effect of herbal drug Withania somnifera on adjuvant induced arthritis in rats, Indian J Exp Biol, 1988, 26, 877-882.

63. Quiney C, Billard C, Mirshahi P, Hyperforin inhibits MMP-9 secreation by B-CLL cells and microtubule formation by endothelial cells, Leukemia, 2006, 20, 583-589.

64. Sagar SM, Yance D, Wong RK, Natural health products that inhibit angiogenesis: a potential source for investigational new agents to treat cancer-Part 1, Curr Oncol, 2006, 13, 14-26.

65. Hu Y, Sun CY, Huang J, Antimyeloma effects of resveratrol through inhibition of angiogenesis, Chin Med J (Engl), 2007, 120, 1672-1677.

66. Kessler JH, Mullauer FB, Roob de GM, Medema J P, Broad *in vitro* efficacy of plant-derived betulinic acid against cell lines derived from the most prevalent human cancer types, Cancer Letters, 2007, 251, 132–145.

CHAPTER 5

VARIOUS OCULAR DRUG DELIVERY SYSTEMS

The Anatomy and Physiology of the Eye

The human eye is the essential sense organ of the body and its anatomy is quite complex. Eye is able to refract light and produce a focused image that can stimulate nervous system and enable the ability to see [1]. The structure of the eye and different parts of the eye are **(Figure 5.1)**:

1. **Aqueous Humour:** It is a jelly-like substance located in the anterior chamber of the eye.

2. **Choroid:** The choroid layer is located behind the retina and absorbs unused radiation.

3. **Ciliary Muscle:** The ciliary muscle is a ring-shaped muscle attached to the iris. It is important because contraction and relaxation of the ciliary muscle controls the shape of the lens.

4. **Cornea:** Cornea is a clear transparent epithelial membrane. Light rays pass through the cornea to reach the retina. The cornea is convex anteriorly and is involved in refracting (bending) light rays to focus them on the retina.

5. **Fovea:** The fovea is a small depression (approx. 1.5 mm in diameter) in the retina. This is the part of the retina in which high-resolution vision of fine detail is possible.

6. **Hyaloid:** The hyaloid diaphragm divides the aqueous humour from the vitreous humour.

7. **Iris:** The iris is the visible coloured part of the eye and extends anteriorly from the ciliary body, lying behind the cornea and in front of the lens. It divides the anterior segment of the eye into anterior and posterior chambers which contain aqueous fluid secreted by the ciliary body. The iris is supplied by parasympathetic and sympathetic nerves. Parasympathetic stimulation constricts the pupil and sympathetic stimulation dilates it.

8. **Lens:** The lens of the eye is a flexible unit that consists of layers of tissue enclosed in a tough capsule. It is suspended from the ciliary muscles by the zonule fibers.

9. **Optic Nerve:** The optic nerve is the second cranial nerve and is responsible for vision. Each nerve contains approximately one million fibres transmitting information from the rod and cone cells of the retina.

10. **Papilla:** The papilla is also known as the "blind spot" and is located at the position from which the optic nerve leaves the retina.

11. **Pupil:** The pupil is the aperture through which light pan and hence the images we see and "perceive" - enters the eye. This is formed by the iris. As the size of the iris increases (or decreases) the size of the pupil decreases (or increases) correspondingly.

12. **Retina:** The retina may be described as the "screen" on which an image is formed by light that has passed into the eye via the cornea, aqueous humour, pupil, lens, then the hyaloid and finally the vitreous humour before reaching the retina. The retina contains photosensitive elements (called rods and cones) that convert the light they detect into nerve impulses that are then sent onto the brain along the optic nerve.

13. **Sclera:** The sclera is a tough white sheath around the outside of the eye-ball. It consists of a membrane that maintains the shape of the eye and gives the attachment to the extrinsic muscle of the eye.

14. **Vitreous Humour:** The vitreous humour (vitreous body) is a jelly-like substance.

Anterior chamber

Pupil

Cornea

Conjunctiva

Iris

Canal of schlemm

Posterior chamber

Zonule

Ciliary body

Choroid

Retina

Sclera

Retina

Choroid

Sclera

Vortex vein

Retinal arterioles and veins

Optic disk

Optic nerve

Central Retinal Artery and vein

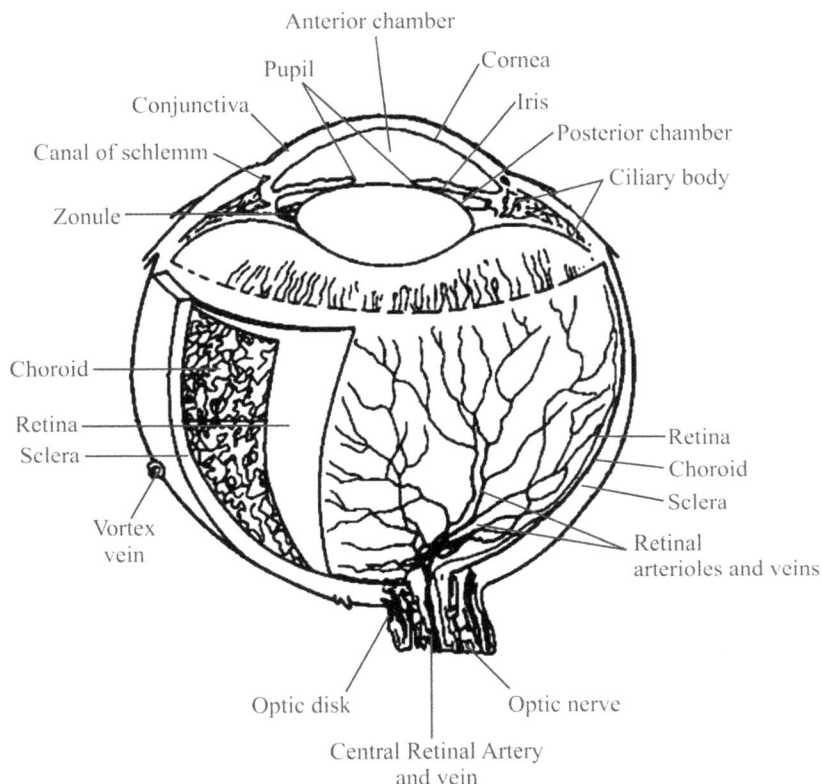

Fig. 5.1 Schematic diagram of the human eye.

Conventional Ocular Drug Delivery Constraints, Ocular Barriers and Pharmacokinetics in the Eye

1. Tear fluid–eye barriers

Most ocular drugs are applied locally as eye drops. However, due to lacrimal drainage and the systemic absorption in the conjunctiva, only a small fraction of the drug is absorbed into the eye[2-3]. After the topical administration of a drug to the ocular surface, there are two main pathways of drug entry into the anterior chamber: via the cornea and via the conjunctiva, the later route being of minor relevance for most drugs. Small and lipophilic molecules (i.e. most clinically used drugs) are absorbed via the cornea, whereas large and hydrophilic molecules (e.g. new potential biotech-drugs such as protein and peptide drugs, gene medicines) are preferably absorbed through the conjunctiva and sclera[4-5].

2.   Cornea

The cornea is an important mechanical and chemical barrier, which limits the access of exogenous substances into the eye and protects the intraocular tissues. The cornea is a clear and vascular structure with average diameter and thickness of 12 mm and 520 mm, respectively[6]. The human cornea consists of five layers: corneal epithelium, basement membrane, Bowman's layer, stroma, Descemet's membrane and endothelium[7]. The corneal epithelium is composed of two to three cell layers of flattened superficial cells, two to three cell layers of wing cells, and a single layer of columnar basal cells. The superficial cells adhere to one another via desmosomes and the cells are encircled by tight junctions[8]. Due to these tight junctions the corneal epithelium represents the rate limiting barrier for the permeation of hydrophilic drugs, whereas the stroma and endothelium offer very little resistance to transcorneal permeation[9-10]. The stroma which constitutes 85–90% of the total corneal mass is mainly composed of hydrated collagen. It exerts a diffusional barrier only to highly lipophilic drugs due to its hydrophilic nature. The corneal endothelial monolayer maintains an effective barrier between the stroma and aqueous humor. Active ion and fluid transport mechanisms in the endothelium are responsible for maintaining corneal transparency[11]. The passive permeability of a drug across the cornea is influenced by various factors, such as the lipophilicity, molecular weight, charge, and degree of ionization of the drug. It was shown that increasing molecular size of the permeating substance decreases the rate of paracellular permeation[12]. The pore size in the intercellular space is an important factor influencing paracellular permeation of drugs. Only relatively small molecules can permeate through the pores, which have an average diameter of 2.0 nm in the rabbit. As the pores of the corneal epithelium are negatively charged at physiological pH, negatively charged molecules permeate slower than positively charged and neutral molecules[13]. Positive charge may decrease the permeation in some cases as well (e.g. cationic aminoPEGs)[14]. This is probably due to ionic interaction between the positively charged molecules and the negatively charged carboxylic groups of tight junction proteins. Lipophilic drugs permeate faster and to a greater extent through the cornea by the transcellular way, the main route of ocular absorption for clinically used drugs. For example, the permeability coefficient (P_{app}) of the lipophilic beta-blocker betaxolol (log D 1.59 (pH 7.4); P_{app} 2.7 × 10^{-5} cm/s) was 25 times higher than the permeability coefficient of the hydrophilic atenolol with similar molecular size (log D × 1.77 (pH 7.4); P_{app} 1.1 × 10^{-6} cm/s) in the isolated rabbit cornea[15-16]. After crossing the cornea the drug diffuses into the aqueous humor and to the anterior uvea. Locally applied drugs that enter the eye via the corneal route cannot reach the retina and vitreous at sufficient therapeutic concentrations[17]. For instance, 30 min after eyedrop administration the concentration of timolol in the vitreous humor was about 26 times lower than the concentration in the aqueous humor[18].

3. Conjunctiva

The conjunctiva is a mucous membrane consisting of an epithelium, which is two to three cell layers thick, and an underlying vascularised connective tissue. It covers the anterior surface of the sclera (bulbar conjunctiva), and is folded at the fornix (fornix conjunctiva) to form the palpebral conjunctiva, which lines the inner surfaces of the eyelids. The conjunctival epithelium plays an important role as protective barrier on the ocular surface, and it contributes to the maintenance of the tear film by the production of mucus glycoproteins. On the apical surface of the epithelium tight junctions are present. The bulbar conjunctiva represents the first barrier for the permeation of topically applied drugs into the eye via the non-corneal route. This route of intraocular entry is relevant for large and hydrophilic substances, which are poorly absorbed through the cornea[19]. It was shown in the rabbit that the conjunctival epithelium has 2 times larger pores and a 16 times higher pore density than the corneal epithelium, which results in a 15- to 25-fold higher permeability in comparison to the cornea. A significant portion of the drug is lost to the systemic circulation while crossing the conjunctiva (**Figure 5.2**)[20-22]. This non-productive absorption is the main reason for the poor bioavailability of drugs entering the eye via the conjunctival/scleral pathway. The remaining drug can diffuse through the sclera, which consists mainly of collagen and mucopolysaccharides, and, in contrast to the conjunctiva, is only poorly vascularised. The sclera is about 10 times more permeable than the cornea and half as permeable as the conjunctiva. The drug can enter the posterior part of the eye (uveal tract, retina, choroid, vitreous humor) using this route.

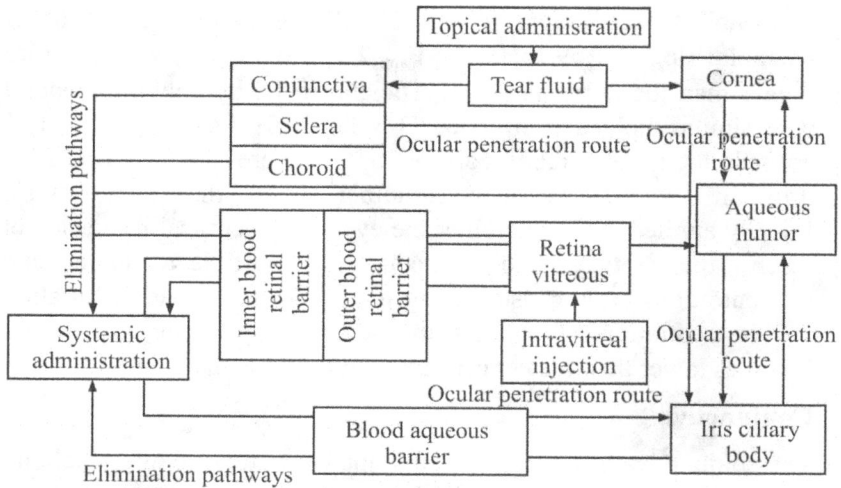

Fig. 5.2 Ocular penetration and elimination route after topical,
systemic and intravitreal route.

4.   Blood–ocular barriers

The establishment and maintenance of therapeutically relevant drug
concentrations in the retina and the vitreous usually require either
systemic or intravitreal drug administration. Systemic application by
oral or intravenous administration has the disadvantage that high
doses of the drug have to be administered, since only a very small
fraction of the drug reaches ocular tissues due to the limited blood
flow and the blood–ocular barriers. The remainder of the drug is
distributed in the entire body leading to unwanted side effects. The
blood–ocular barrier can be overcome by the intravitreal injection of
drugs, but this route of administration is associated with several
problems, including risks of endophthalmitis, damage to lens or
retinal detachment, and low patient compliance[23]. There are two
blood–ocular barrier systems in the eye: the blood–aqueous barrier
and the blood–retinal barrier, which provide a controlled
environment for the internal ocular tissues.

(a)   Blood–aqueous barrier

The blood–aqueous barrier (BAB) is located in the anterior part
of the eye. It is formed by endothelial cells of the blood vessels
in the iris, and the non-pigmented cell layer of the ciliary
epithelium. Tight junctional complexes are present in both cell
layers. These cell layers prevent non-specific passage of solutes
into the intraocular milieu that might otherwise negatively

influence transparency and chemical equilibrium of the ocular fluids[24]. However, even when the BAB is intact, its barrier function is not complete. For instance, whereas injected horse radish peroxidase (HRP, molecular mass 40 kDa) cannot pass through the iris blood vessels, it can permeate through the fenestrated capillaries of the ciliary processes, and reach the aqueous humor[25-26]. This permeability accounts for the presence of low levels of plasma proteins in the aqueous humor. The outward movement of substances from the aqueous humor across the iris blood vessels into systemic circulation is less restricted[27]. The iris tissue itself is porous, and drugs dissolved in the aqueous humor can freely enter across its anterior surface. Some drugs are then absorbed by the iris pigments or they are removed from the anterior chamber by passage into the iris blood vessels. Especially, small and lipophilic drugs can enter the uveal blood circulation via the blood–aqueous barrier and they are consequently eliminated more rapidly from the anterior chamber than larger and more hydrophilic drugs, which are eliminated by aqueous humor turnover only[28]. For instance, the clearance of pilocarpine was determined to be 13.0 ml/min, whereas the clearance of inulin was close to the rate of aqueous humor turnover[29-30]. Although aqueous humor turnover, which is 3.0–4.7 ml/min in rabbits and 2.0–3.0 ml/min in humans[31], is often considered to be the major route of drug elimination from the anterior chamber, many drugs have clearance values exceeding the rate of aqueous humor turnover, which indicates the presence of alternative elimination pathways.

(b) Blood–retinal barrier

The blood–retinal barrier (BRB) is located in the posterior part of the eye. It is formed by the endothelial cells of retinal blood vessels (inner blood–retinal barrier) and the retinal pigment epithelial cells (outer blood–retinal barrier). The multilayered neural retina is separated by the subretinal space from the retinal pigment epithelium (RPE) monolayer, which separates the outer surface of the neural retina from the choroid. Under physiologic conditions the retina is firmly attached to the RPE. The RPE plays a vital role in maintaining the viability and function of the neural retina[32]. The RPE is, for example, responsible for the removal of fluid from the subretinal space in order to maintain retinal adhesion and to keep the neural retina in a state of dehydration. Because of its tight junctions the RPE forms a strong barrier, but it is capable of a number of specialized transport processes. Only selected nutrients are exchanged between choroid and retina, the transcellular and paracellular passage of other molecules across the RPE is restricted. Because of their specialized functions the RPE cells have unique morphologic and functional polarity properties. One feature of RPE cells is the predominant apical localization of Na^+-K^+-ATPase, which regulates intracellular Na^+ and K^+ homeostasis[33]. Apart from forming the blood–retinal barrier, the RPE has several other functions, such as the phagocytosis of the outer segments shed by retinal rods and cones; transport of nutrients and metabolic products; retinoid transport and metabolism; the absorption of light and the dissipation of heat energy derived from incident light; synthesis of enzymes, growth factors and pigments; and participation in the immune reactivity of the retina. The inner blood–retinal barrier is constituted by endothelial cells, which cover the lumen of retinal capillaries and separate the retinal tissue and the blood. The retinal endothelial cells have intercellular tight junctions. Glial cells (astrocytes and muller cells) are in contact with the vessel walls and provide signals which induce barrier properties in the endothelial cells[34]. Due to these tight junctions the paracellular transport of compounds is restricted. In these respects the inner blood–retinal barrier is similar to the blood–brain barrier, which is constituted by the endothelial cells of the microvessels in the brain, pericytes and astrocytes. While the density of tight junctions and cytoplasmic vesicles was determined to be higher in retinal vessels than in the brain, pericytes are 4 times as numerous in the retina, which probably compensates for the more permeable endothelial barrier[35]. Stewart and Tuor determined with a vascular tracer that transfer by passive diffusion is about 4 times higher in the retina than in the brain of rats. As the blood–retinal barrier prevents entrance of toxic molecules, plasma components and water into the retina, it restricts the passage of systemically applied drugs as well. After systemic administration the concentration of a drug in the vitreous is typically only 1–2% of the concentration in the plasma. Permeability coefficients across isolated porcine RPE tissue sheets varied from 10^{-7} cm/s for poorly permeable molecules, such as the hydrophilic beta-blocker atenolol, to 10^{-5} cm/s for highly permeable substances, such as memantine and nicotine[36]. The permeability coefficient of sodium fluorescein (1.81×10^{-7} cm/s) determined with this model was found to be in the *in vivo* range. Like the RPE, also retinal vessel walls are poorly permeable to proteins (e.g. horse radish peroxidase) and small hydrophilic compounds (e.g. sodium fluorescein), whereas lipophilic substances can permeate retinal capillary endothelial cells more easily. Many substances are eliminated from the vitreous body either by active transport or passive diffusion across the BRB. This is highly relevant in intravitreal drug administration, since high lipophilicity of the drug or the presence of an active transport mechanism lead to a rapid transport from the vitreous across the retina into the systemic blood circulation. A longer half-life in the vitreous can be observed when the passage of the drug through the BRB is not possible, and the drug has to diffuse into the anterior chamber first to be removed either by aqueous blood-flow or after diffusion across the iris surface. For example, after intravitreal injection the rate of loss of gentamicin, which is removed from the vitreous via the anterior chamber, is about 0.035 h^{-1} in the rabbit, where as for penicillin, which leaves the eye by crossing the retina, the rate of loss is 0.18 h^{-1}, so that the half-life of penicillin in the vitreous is 5 times shorter than the half-life of gentamicin.

Formulation Approaches to Improve Ocular Bioavailability

Various approaches that have been attempted to increase the bioavailability and the duration of therapeutic action of ocular drugs can be divided into two categories. The first is based on use of the drug delivery systems, which provide the controlled and continuous delivery of ophthalmic drugs. The second involves, minimizing precorneal drug loss. Some of the requisites of controlled ocular delivery systems are:

1. To overcome the side effects of pulsed dosing produced by conventional systems.

2. To provide sustained and controlled drug delivery.

3. To increase ocular bioavailability of drug by increasing corneal contact time.

4. To provide targeting within the ocular globes so as to prevent the loss to other ocular sites.

5. To circumvent the protective barriers like drainage, lacrimation and diversion of exogenous chemicals into systemic circulation by conjunctiva.

6. To provide comfort and compliance to the patient and yet improve the therapeutic performance of the drug over conventional systems.

7. To provide better housing of the delivery system in the eye so that the loss to other tissues besides cornea is prevented.

1. Viscous Solutions and Hydrogels

Viscous solutions and hydrogels, based upon the addition of hydrocolloids to simpler aqueous solutions, are the most common formulations. There is no clear-cut frontier between very viscous solutions and gels in terms of biopharmaceutical results. However, preformed gels are administered in the same way as an ointment, which is less convenient for the patient than the instillation of a viscous drop. The most common polymers used in viscous solutions are cellulose derivatives, carbomers, polysaccharides, and, recently, hyaluronic acid. The advantage offered by this last product could be dependent upon the active ingredient and the formulation environment[37]. Polyvinyl alcohol and polyvinyl pyrolidone are also used in ophthalmic drugs. Gels permit longer residence time in the precorneal area than viscous solutions. This has encouraged researchers to work on formulations that would be (viscous) solutions in the drug vials but would gel in the conjunctival cul-de-sac. Three main mechanisms have been explored to induce the sol/gel transition in the conjunctival pouch, namely a change in pH, a change in temperature, or a change in ionic environment[38]. Eventually one formulation of timolol, which was based on gellan gum that underwent a sol/gel transition due to the ionic content of the tears, reached the market in 1994 (Timoptic XE)[39-40]. Phase transition systems are liquid dosage forms which shift to gel or solid phase when instilled in the cul-de-sac. Polymers like Lutrol FC-127, Poloxamer-407[41] whose viscosity increases when its temperature is raised to 37 °C. In situ forming gels have been actively pursued. Product(s) using the gellan gum technology[42] with polymer associations like those reported by Kumar et al., 1994[43], Smart Geltechnology[44] are examples of technologies that use this approach. This field of intricately entangled polymers seems promising since new "patentable" entities might be obtained through in-depth studies of associations of well-established products. The aqueous formulations of such mixtures exhibit changes in physical properties, i.e. sol-gel transformation, with changes in the environment, e.g. temperature, pH, or ionic strength.

2. Bioadhesives

It offer several advantages like localizing a dosage form within a particular region, increasing drug bioavailability, promoting contact with surface for longer time, reduce dosage frequency. Several synthetic and natural polymers are used for this purpose like sodium hyaluronate, chondroitin sulphate (natural polymers) and various polyacrylate, carbopols (synthetic polymers). A good bioadhesive should exhibit a near zero contact angle to allow maximum contact with the mucin coat[45].

3. Soft contact lenses

The rationale for corneal contact devices has not been fully explored in therapy. It is generally accepted that soft contact lenses can act as a reservoir for drugs, providing improved release of the therapeutic agent. Presoaked lenses are considered a more efficient and reliable delivery system. Imprinted soft contact lenses are promising drug devices able to provide greater and more sustained drug concentrations in tear fluid with lower doses than conventional eye drops[46].

5. Ocular iontophoresis

Iontophoresis is a process by which the direct current drives ions into cell or tissues. Antibiotics, antifungals have been tried by this method[47]. Recent progress in the technology of the associated hardware has stimulated interest in a renewal of its use in ophthalmology.

6. Collagen shields

Friedburg *et al.* (1991)[48] developed collagen shields to promote wound healing and perhaps more importantly to deliver a variety of medications to the cornea and other ocular tissues. For drug delivery, the shields are rehydrated in aqueous solution of the drug where by the drug is absorbed by the protein matrix and is released once the shield dissolves in the eye. However, their size and the constraints they impose on vision render them impractical for a new drug delivery system. Suspensions of collagen microparticulates accepted[49].

7. Pseudolatices

These are a new class of polymeric colloidal dispersion and film forming agents used for topical applications into the animals and human beings for sustaining the drug activity *in vivo*[50].

8. Ocular penetration enhancer

Penetration enhancers like actin filament inhibitors; surfactants, bile salts, etc. have been used to increase the bioavailability of topically applied proteins and peptides[51].

9. Ocular inserts and implants

Various erodible implants marketed to date like Lacrisert, Soluble ocular drug insert are made of mainly collagen, fibrin, HPMC, etc. Two products Alza Ocusert[52] and Merck Lacrisert have been marketed, although Ocusert is no longer sold. Ocusert was an insoluble delicate sandwich technology. Filled with sufficient pilocarpine for 1 week's use, where as Lacrisert is a soluble minirod of hydroxypropyl cellulose, nonmedicated and dissolving within 24 h to treat dry-eye syndromes. Other inserts are more like implants to be placed in the eye tissues by surgery.

10. Dispersed Systems

Dispersed systems based on liposomes, nanoparticles, or nanocapsules have been extensively studied for potential ophthalmic use[53-54]. The development of marketable products based on these nano products has been very challenging and a definitive technology has not yet been established. The major issues for this type of delivery system include: percentage of dispersed phase/entrapment coefficient problem (i.e., how much of the active ingredient will be present in a drop of the final product), stability and shelf life, antimicrobial preservation, tolerance of the used surfactants, and, last but not least, large-scale manufacture of sterile preparations. Nanosized systems based on liposomes, nanoparticles, and nanocapsules have been extensively studied and published and call the ophthalmic formulator's attention. Beyond the problem of the entrapment percentage of the active pharmaceutical ingredient, the retention of these particles in the conjunctival pouch is a key consideration. This retention must be effective in providing an extended source of active and to allow the drug to leak out from the dispersed phase before the instilled formulation is drained away from the precorneal area. Positively charged liposomes were described to have a greater affinity for ocular tissues[55]. A possible vehicle to administer these delicate nanosystems could be a gel, as was described for liposomes[56]. Microemulsions might be systems of future interest, with the basic caveats concerning sterile manufacturing, long-term stability, patient tolerance with any surfactant, and the difficulty to adequately preserve a biphasic system. Pilocarpine was described to largely benefit from such a formulation, and cyclosporine is a potential candidate for it[57]. The advantges and disadvantages of various approaches are shown in **Table 5.1.**

Table 5.1 Various noninvasive ocular drug delivery approaches.

Delivery system	Advantages	Disadvantages
Aqueous suspension	Best for drugs with slow dissolution	Rapid loss
Viscosity imparting agent	Increased residence time and exhibit pseudoplastic flow	Problem in flowability and dispensing
Prodrug and Ion pairs	Useful for poorly absorable drugs, penetrates the corneal epithelium faster, better transfer across cornea by associated ions	Dependa on biochemical and metabolic consideration of the eye and physicochemical properties of the drug
Ointments	Bioavailabilty is higher than aqueous solution or suspension, flexibility in drug choice, improved drug stability, once daily application, increased contact time	No true sustaining effect, blurred vision, drug choice limited by partition coefficient
Gels	Comfortable, less blurred vision than ointment	No rate control on diffusion, matted eyelids after use
In-situ gelling system	Administerd like eye drops, comfortable, less blurred vision	No rate control on diffusion
Non-erodible insert	Zero order drug release, long delivery time, flexibility for type of drug selected	Difficulaty in handling, nonbiodegradable, costly, foreign body sensation
Erodible inserts	Flexibility in drug type and dissolution rate, need only to be introduced into the eye and not removed	Patient discomfort, requires patient insertion, movement of system around the eye, occasional product discharge

Table 5.1 *Contd...*

Delivery system	Advantages	Disadvantages
Liposomes	Resistance to drainage, biocompatible and biodegradable, patient acceptance, increased residence time	Possible oil entrapment, unstable due to hydrolysis, limited drug loading, costly
Nanoparticles	Patient acceptance, useful to deliver lipophilic drug	Not suitable for water soluble drugs
Nanogels	Patient acceptance, Resistance to drainage, biocompatible and biodegradable, patient acceptance, increased residence time	Less blurred vision

References

1. www.wepediafreecyclopedia.com.

2. Lee VH and Robinson JR, Mechanistic and quantitative evaluation of precorneal pilocarpine disposition in albino rabbits, J Pharm Sci, 1979, 68, 673–684.

3. Maurice DM and Mishima S, Ocular pharmacokinetics, in: M.L. Sears (Ed.), Handbook of Experimental Pharmacology, vol. 69. Pharmacology of the Eye, Springer, Berlin, 1984, pp. 16–119.

4. Ahmed TFP, Importance of the noncorneal absorption route in topical ophthalmic drug delivery, Invest Ophthalmol Vis Sci, 1985, 26, 584–587.

5. Schoenwald RD and Huang HS, Corneal penetration behaviour of beta-blocking agents I: physicochemical factors, J Pharm Sci, 1983, 72, 1266–1272.

6. Chastain JE, General considerations in ocular drug delivery, in: A.K. Mitra (Ed.), Ophthalmic Drug Delivery Systems, Marcel Dekker, New York, 2003, pp. 59–107.

7. Young B and Heath JW, Wheater's Functional Histology, Harcourt Publishers Ltd, Edinburgh, 2000. pp. 382–393.

8. Klyce SD and Crosson CE, Transport processes across the rabbit corneal epithelium: a review, Curr Eye Res, 1985, 4, 323–331.

9. Huang HS, Schoenwald RD, Lach JL, Corneal penetration behavior of beta-blocking agents II: assessment of barrier contributions, J Pharm Sci, 1983, 72, 1272–1279.

10. Huang AJ, Tseng SC, Kenyon KR, Paracellular permeability of corneal and conjunctival epithelia, Invest Ophthalmol Vis Sci, 1989, 30, 684–689.

11. Sunkara G and Kompella UB, Membrane transport processes in the eye, in: A.K. Mitra (Ed.), Ophthalmic Drug Delivery Systems, Marcel Dekker, New York, 2003, pp. 17–58.

12. Ha¨ma¨la¨inen KM, Kananen K, Auriola S, Kontturi K, Urtti A, Characterization of paracellular and aqueous penetration routes in cornea, conjunctiva, and sclera, Invest Ophthalmol Vis Sci, 1997, 38, 627–634.

13. Rojanasakul Y and Robinson JR, Transport mechanisms of the cornea: characterization of barrier permselectivity, Int J Pharm, 1989, 55, 237–246.

14. Palmgre'n JJ, Toropainen E, Auriola S, Urtti A, Liquid chromatographic–electrospray ionization mass spectrometric analysis of neutral and charged polyethylene glycols, J Chromatogr A, 2002, 976, 165–170.

15. Wang W, Sasaki H, Chien DS, Lee VH, Lipophilicity influence on conjunctival drug penetration in the pigmented rabbit: a comparison with corneal penetration, Curr Eye Res, 1991, 10, 571–579.

16. M.R. Prausnitz, J.S. Noonan, Permeability of cornea, sclera, and conjunctiva: a literature analysis for drug delivery to the eye, J. Pharm. Sci. 87 (1998) 1479–1488.

17. S. Duvvuri, S. Majumdar, A.K. Mitra, Drug delivery to the retina: challenges and opportunities, Expert Opin. Biol. Ther. 3 (2003) 45–56.

18. Urtti, J.D. Pipkin, G. Rork, T. Sendo, U. Finne, A.J. Repta, Controlled drug delivery devices for experimental ocular studies with timolol 2. Ocular and systemic absorption in rabbits, Int. J. Pharm. 61 (1990) 241–249.

19. Ahmed, The noncorneal route in ocular drug delivery, in: A.K. Mitra (Ed.), Ophthalmic Drug Delivery Systems, Marcel Dekker, New York, 2003, pp. 335–363.

20. Salminen UL, Concentration-dependent precorneal loss of pilocarpine in rabbit eyes, Acta Ophthalmol, 1985, 63, 502–506.

21. Chang SC and Lee VH, Nasal and conjunctival contributions to the systemic absorption of topical timolol in the pigmented rabbit:

implications in the design of strategies to maximize the ratio of ocular to systemic absorption, J Ocul Pharmacol, 1987, 3, 159–169.

22. Salminen UL, Minimizing systemic absorption of topically administered ophthalmic drugs, Surv Ophthalmol, 1993, 37, 435–456.

23. Couvreur BP and Fattal E, Intravitreal administration of antisense oligonucleotides: potential of liposomal delivery, Prog Retin Eye Res, 2000, 19, 131–147.

24. Cunha-Vaz JG, The blood–ocular barriers: past, present, and future, Doc Ophthalmol, 1997, 93, 149–157.

25. Barsotti MF, Bartels SP, Freddo TF, Kamm RD, The source of protein in the aqueous humor of the normal monkey eye, Invest Ophthalmol Vis Sci, 1992, 33, 581–595.

26. Schlingemann RO, Hofman P, Klooster J, Blaauwgeers HG, Van der Gaag R, Vrensen GF, Ciliary muscle capillaries have blood–tissue barrier characteristics, Exp Eye Res, 1998, 66, 747–754.

27. Jumbe NL and Miller MH, Ocular drug transfer following systemic drug administration, in: A.K. Mitra (Ed.), Ophthalmic Drug Delivery Systems, Marcel Dekker, New York, 2003, pp. 109–133.

28. Salminen UL, Animal pharmacokinetic studies, in: A.K. Mitra (Ed.), Ophthalmic Drug Delivery Systems, Marcel Dekker, New York, 1993, pp. 121–136.

29. Conrad JM and Robinson JR, Aqueous chamber drug distribution volume measurement in rabbits, J Pharm Sci, 1977, 66, 219–224.

30. Schoenwald RD, Ocular pharmacokinetics and pharmacodynamics, in: A.K. Mitra (Ed.), Ophthalmic Drug Delivery Systems, Marcel Dekker, New York, 2003, pp. 135–179.

31. Worakul N and Robinson JR, Ocular pharmacokinetics/pharmacodynamics, Eur J Pharm Biopharm, 1997, 44, 71–83.

32. Marmor MF, Structure function and disease of the retinal pigment epithelium,, in: M.F. Marmor, T.J. Wolfensberger (Eds.), The Retinal Pigment Epithelium, Oxford University Press, New York, 1998, pp. 3–9.

33. Quinn RH and Miller SS, Ion transport mechanisms in native human retinal pigment epithelium, Invest Ophthalmol Vis Sci, 1992, 33, 3513–3527.

34. Gardner TW, Antonetti DA, Barber AJ, Lieth E, Tarbell JA, The molecular structure and function of the inner blood–retinal barrier, Doc Ophthalmol, 1999, 97, 229–237.

35. Stewart PA and Tuor UI, Blood–eye barriers in the rat: correlation of ultrastructure with function, J Comp Neurol, 1994, 340, 566–576.

36. Steuer H, Jaworski A, Stoll D, Schlosshauer B, In vitro model of the outer blood–retina barrier, Brain Res Brain Res Protoc, 2004, 13, 26–36.

37. Bernatchez SF, Camber O, Tabatabay C, Gurny R, Use of hyaluronic acid. P Edman, Biopharmaceutics of Ocular Drug Delivery, Boca Raton, FL: CRC Press, 1993, 105–120.

38. Gurny R, Ibrahim H, Buri P, The development and use of in situ formed gels, triggered by pH. P. Edman, Biopharmaceutics of Ocular Drug Delivery, Boca Raton, FL: CRC Press, 1993, 81–90.

39. Rozier A, Mazuel C, Grove J, Plazonnet B, Gelrite: a novel, ion activated, in-situ gelling polymer for ophthalmic vehicles: effect on bioavailability of timolol, Int J Pharm, 1989, 57, 163–168.

40. Vogel R, Kulaga SF, Laurenc JK, Gross RL, Haik BG, Karp D, Koby M, Zimmerman TJ, The effect of a Gelrite vehicle on the efficacy of low concentration of timolol, Invest Ophthalmol Vis Sci, 1990, 31: 404.

41. Miller SC and Donovan MD, Effect of poloxamer 407 gel on the miotic activity of pilocarpine nitrate in rabbits, Int J Pharm, 1982, 12, 147.

42. Merck and Co, 1989. US patent 4, 861,760.

43. Kumar S, Haglund BO, Himmelstein KJ, In situ–forming gels for ophthalmic drug delivery, J Ocul Pharmacol, 1994, 10, 47–56.

44. Ron ES, Smart Gel: A new thermogelling polymer mixture for drug delivery, Proc Sci, 1996, 22, 220–227.

45. Robinson JR and Mlynek GM, Bioadhesive and phase-change polymers for ocular drug delivery, Adv Drug Del Rev, 1995, 16, 45–50.

46. Haruyuki H, Akihito F, Yuka T, Yuri M, Carmen AL, Ocular release of timolol from molecularly imprinted soft contact lenses, Biomaterials, 2005, 26, 1293-1298.

47. Hughes L and Maurice D, A fresh look at iontophoresis, Arch Ophthalmol, 1984, 102, 1825-1829.

48. Friedberg ML, Pleyer U and Mondino BJ, Device drug delivery to the eye. Collagen shields, iontophoresis, and pumps, Ophthalmol, 1991, 98, 725–732.

49. Kaufman HE, Steinemann TL, Lehman E, Thompson HW, Varnell ED, Jacob Labarre JT, Gebhardt BM, Collagen-based drug delivery and artifcial tears, J Ocul Pharmacol, 1994, 10, 17–27.

50. Vyas SP, Ramchandraiah S, Jain CP and Jain SK, Polymeric pseudolatices bearing pilocarpine for controlled ocular delivery, J Microencap, 1992, 9, 347-355.

51. Rojanasakul Y, Paddock SW, Robinson JR, Confocal laser scanning microscopic examination of transport pathways and barriers of some peptides across the cornea, Int J Pharm, 1990, 61, 163.

52. Urquhart J, Development of Ocusert pilocarpine ocular therapeutic systems. Robinson JR, Ophthalmic Drug Delivery Systems, Washington, DC: American Pharmaceutical Association, 1980, 105–108.

53. Gurny R, Boye T, Ibrahim H, Ocular therapy with nanoparticulate systems for controlled drug delivery, J Control Rel 1985, 2, 353–36.

54. Lee VHL, Urrea PT, Smith RE, Schauzun DJ, Ocular drug bioavailability from topically applied liposomes, Surv Ophthalmol, 1985, 29, 335–348.

55. Schaeffer HE and Krohn DL, Liposomes in topical drug delivery, Invest Ophthal Vis Pharmacol, 1982, 10, 17–27.

56. Bochot A, Fattal E, Grossiord JL, Puisieux F, Couvreur P, Characterization of a new ocular delivery system based on a dispersion of liposomes in a thermosensitive gel, Int J Pharm, 1998, 162, 119–127.

57. Naveh N, Muchtar S, Benita S, Pilocarpine incorporated into a submicron emulsion vehicle causes an unexpectedly prolonged ocular hypotensive effect in rabbits, J Ocul Pharmacol, 1994, 10, 509–520.

CHAPTER 6

NOVEL STRATEGIES FOR THE TREATMENT OF DIABETIC RETINOPATHY

Noval Drug Delivery Systems

There are various noval drug delivery systems such as liposomes, microemulsions, nanosuspension, micellar systems, nanoparticles, dendrimers, viral vectors and nanocrystals.

1. Liposomes

Liposomes are spherical vesicles that are prepared using one or more amphiphilic phospholipids (such as phosphatidylcholine) and cholesterol that self-associate into bilayers that have aqueous interior. Liposomes may be formulated into small structures (80–100 nm) that encapsulate either hydrophilic drug in the aqueous interior or lipophilic within the lipid bilayers. Drug release, *in vivo* stability and biodistribution are determined by the size, surface charge, surface hydrophobicity and membrane fluidity[1]. Liposomes have low toxicity based on selection of components that are safe and application of processes that are not damaging to the drug. Some of the other benefits for liposomes in drug delivery are as follows: (i) they are versatile in size, (ii) composition and (iii) bilayer fluidity and (iv) they are capable of displaying drugs on their surface or encapsulating drugs within the bilayer. Examples of lipids that are used to prepare liposomes are dioleylpropyl trimethylammonium chloride (DOTMA); dioleoyl trimethylammonium propane (DOTAP) and dimethylaminoethane carbamoyl cholestrerol.

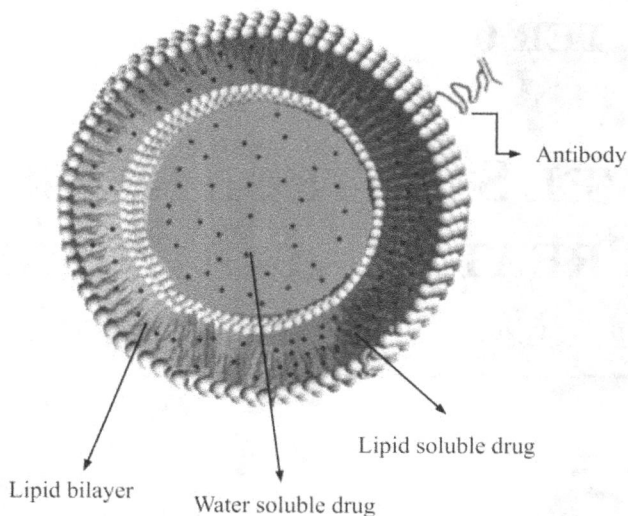

Antibody

Lipid soluble drug

Lipid bilayer

Water soluble drug

Fig. 6.1 Structure of liposome.

Liposomes were also evaluated in an attempt to improve bioavailability of ophthalmic drugs after topical instillation, because they are stable, biocompatible and biodegradable liquid preparations. Depending on the method of preparation, vesicles of various structure (multilamellar, small unilamellar, large unilamellar, oligolamellar vesicles) and size are obtained, which can influence the pharmacokinetics of the drug[2]. The potential of liposomes in ocular drug delivery is limited by their rapid clearance from the precorneal area, low encapsulation efficiency, rapid leakage (premature release) of incorporated drug into the blood, poor stability and high cost of production at an industrial scale. In order to delay or prevent interactions with reticuloendothelial systems (RES) liposome formulations have been modified by inclusion of polyethylene glycol (PEG) that serves as a barrier preventing interaction with plasma proteins. The typical diagram of the liposome are shown in **Figure 6.1.**

The same rapid drainage was observed as for aqueous eye drops, especially in the case of neutral liposomes and negatively charged liposomes[3]. Positively charged liposomes on the other hand were reported to exhibit a prolonged precorneal retention, because of electrostatic interaction with the negatively charged corneal epithelium. It is proposed that positively charged liposomes bind intimately on the eye surface, increase the residence time and thus enhance drug absorption. Accumulation of drug in the cornea could occur by endocytosis of the liposomes[4]. In order to enhance adherence to the corneal/conjunctival surface, dispersion of the liposomes in mucoadhesive gels or coating the liposomes with mucoadhesive polymers was proposed. Several mucoadhesive polymers were employed: poly(acrylic acid) (PAA), hyaluronic acid (HA), chitosan, poloxamer. The binding or anchoring of cytoadhesive ligands and lecthins was another strategy investigated. Even if an enhanced precorneal retention was observed with respect to non-coated vesicles and aqueous solution, no significant increase in the bioavailability of the drug was measured on rabbits. This lack of bioavailability-enhancing effect of the PAA coated liposomes was attributed to the tear film pH of 7.4, which is less favourable for mucoadhesion compared to a pH of 5.5. On the other hand, Nagarsenker *et al.* demonstrated that positively charged liposomes loaded with tropicamide and neutral liposomes dispersed in a polycarbophil gel were more effective than neutral liposomes with regard to the duration of drug action (mydriatic response). Durrani et al. investigated the influence of Carbopol 1342 on the bioavailability of liposomes made by the reverse-phase evaporation method (REV) and loaded with pilocarpine. The coating polymer film decreased the drug release *in-vitro*, but *in-vivo*, in rabbits, the coated liposomes caused a significantly prolonged duration of the miotic effect as compared to aqueous solutions and non-coated vesicles[5].

2. Microemulsion

A simplified definition for microemulsions is that they contain two phases consisting of two immiscible liquids that are mixed togather and stabilized with the aid of a surfactant with or without a co-surfactant. Microemulsions are thermodynamically stable fluid, isotropically clear and may have droplets in the range of 5–100 nm. Microemulsions have been proposed as drug delivery systems to enhance the absorption of drug across biological membranes[6]. The application of microemulsions may offer many advantages for marketed pharmaceutical products, such as (i) increased solubility and stability of drugs incorporated in the dispersed phase and (ii) ease and economy of scale-up (since expensive mixing equipment is often not needed). Some of the major drawbacks are (a) premature leakage/release of incorporated drug since drugs are entrapped in droplets; (b) phase inversion which can occur from instability in biological fluids; (c) many effective surfactants and or co-surfactants do not have a pharmaceutically acceptable toxicity profile; and (d) microemulsion systems often require development of complex systems that may be time consuming leading to significantly long product development time lines. Additionally, microemulsions have been used as templates to prepare solid nanoparticles. Solid nanoparticles were cured from microemulsion systems by use of photochemistry[7], polymerization[8], or a sequence of heating and cooling[9].

3. Nanosuspensions

Nanosuspension refers to production of sub-micron-sized particles by subjecting the combination of drug and a suitable emulsifier to the process of milling or high-pressure homogenization. Conventional milling and precipitation processes generally result in particles with sizes that are much greater than 1 mm. As such, a critical step in the nanosuspension preparation is the choice of the manufacturing procedure to ensure production of sub-micron particles. Particle size reduction to sizes below 1 mm is usually difficult due to possible particle aggregation and generation of high surface area materials. Milling techniques that have been used to generate nano-sized particles are ball milling or pearl milling that applies milling beads of sizes ranging from 0.4 to 3 mm. These beads may be composed of glass, ceramics or plastics[10]. The time required for milling depends on the hardness and brittleness of the drug material in comparison to milling material and inertial forces set up within the mill. Some of the challenges that milling processes can pose in drug development are (i) undesirable erosion of the milling equipment components into the drug product; (ii) the process is usually time consuming, thereby prolonging drug development time; (iii) milling over a few days may bring the risk of microbiological problems or increases in the cost of production; also (iv) prolonged milling may induce the formation of amorphous domains in crystalline starting materials or may lead to changes in the polymorphic form of the drug. The generation of amorphous form of the drug is problematic because these forms may crystallize during the shelf life of the drug leaching to changes in solubility and bioavailability of the drug. An example of the conversion of crystalline to amorphous form of the drug was observed in jet milling of albuterol sulfate. Also, the generation of high-energy surfaces that affected wettability was observed with acetylsalicylic acid. Some examples of nano-sized particles produced by milling are (i) naproxen nanoparticles approximately 200 nm in diameter[11] and (ii) danazol particles of a mean size of 169 nm[12]. An example of a commercialized mechanical process for nanoparticle preparation is NanoCrystal technology that was developed and patented in 1992 which is now a platform technology of Elan Drug Technologies. There are four approved drug products in the USA that are based on NanoCrystal technology: (a) Rapamune (sirolimus) tablets by Wyeth; (b) Tricor (fenofibrate) tablets by Abbott; (c) Emend (aprepitant) capsules by Merck; and (d) Megace ES (megestrol) oral suspension by Par Pharmaceuticals[13]. Additionally, production of sub-micron-sized drug particles by high pressure homogenization has been well reported[14]. An example of commercialized high-pressure homogenization process, Dissocubes was developed and patented in 1994. The process has been applied in Skye Pharma's insoluble drug delivery (IDD) and Baxter NanoEdge platforms. These have resulted in some drug products, namely: (i) Triglide (fenofibrate) by SkyePharma based on the IDD technology; (ii) Abrane, an albumin-stabilized nanoparticle formulation of paclitaxel by Abraxis BioScience. Abraxane is approved in the USA as a second-line therapy for breast cancer and in Canada for metastatic breast cancer. The formation of nanosuspensions is based on the cavitation forces created in high-pressure homogenizers such as piston-gap homogenizers. In the process, an aqueous suspension of the drug in surfactant solution is made which is subsequently passed through a high pressure of typically 1500 bar at 3–20 homogenization cycles[15]. The suspension is then passed through a small gap in the homogenizer of typical width 25 mm at 1500 bar. The cavitation forces are built up due to a number of factors such as (i) narrowness of the gap resulting from streaming velocity of the suspension and dynamic fluid pressure increase and (ii) a decrease in static pressure of the fluid and resultant production of water vapor that escapes the homogenization gap. The cavitation forces that are created are strong enough to break drug microparticles to nanoparticles. An example is in the microfluidization of atovaquone to obtain particles in the 100–300 nm size range[16]. In most cases, nanosuspension particles have an average size ranging from 40 to 500 nm with a small (0.1%) proportion of particles larger than 5 mm. For the purpose of large-scale production of drug delivery systems, high-pressure homogenizers are available with different capacities that are suitable for drug development and large-scale manufacturing. A major challenge in the use of high-pressure homogenization is the possible changes in drug crystal structure that can cause batch-to-batch variation in crystallinity level.

4. Nanoparticles

The rationale for the development of various particulate systems for the delivery of ophthalmic drugs was based on possible entrapment of the particles in the ocular mucus layer and the interaction of bioadhesive polymer chains with mucins inducing a prolonged residence, and slow drainage. Furthermore, controlled drug release and enhanced absorption or even endocytosis in the case of nanoparticles should improve bioavailability.

Nanoparticles are solid colloidal particles, ranging in size from 1 to 1000 nm, consisting of various macromolecules in which the therapeutic drugs can be adsorbed, entrapped or covalently attached. Solid nanoparticles offer distinct advantages in drug development which can be ascribed to their physical stability and the possibility of modifying the formulating materials in order to achieve controlled release characteristics. The ability to formulate nanoparticles to achieve sustained release offers an opportunity for product life cycle management by developing formulations with decreased dosing frequency for drugs that are going off patent. There has been a variety of materials used to engineer solid nanoparticles both with and without surface functionality. Perhaps the most widely used are the aliphatic polyesters such as poly(lactic acid) (PLA), the more hydrophilic poly(glycolic acid) (PGA) and their copolymers poly(lactide-coglycolide) (PLGA). The degradation rate of these polymers and often the corresponding drug release rate can vary from days (PGA) to months (PLA). The effectiveness of nanoparticles in drug delivery can be attributed to many factors such as physical and biological stability, good tolerability of the components, simplicity of the manufacturing process, possibility of facile scale-up of the manufacturing process, amenability to freeze drying and sterilization.

Polyalkyl cyanoacrylates (PACA) and polyalkyl methacrylates were most commonly used for the preparation of drug carriers in the size range 200–500 nm. The choice is based on the mucoadhesive or bioadhesive properties of these PAA derivatives. Kreuter confirmed the binding to the cornea and conjunctiva after instillation, while Diepold *et al.* reported higher concentrations of nanoparticles in inflamed compared to healthy rabbit eyes. Many studies were devoted to the improvement of glaucoma therapy, infections and reduction of side effects. Sustained drug release and prolonged therapeutic effect were observed, except when the drug had a high affinity for the polymer. The increased bioavailability was attributed to the bioadhesive properties of polyalkyl cyanoacrylates. The precorneal residence time of PACA nanoparticles could further be increased by incorporation into a poly(ethylene glycol) gel or by coating with poly(ethylene glycol).

(i) Polymeric nanoparticles

Polymeric nanoparticles made with biodegradable polymers have been widely applied in drug delivery. Many FDA-approved biodegradable and biocompatible polymers have been used in nanoparticle preparation. These include polylactide-polyglycolide copolymers, polyacrylates and polycaprolactones. Examples of natural polymers are albumin, gelatin, alginate, collagen and chitosan. Nanoparticles can be prepared from polymerization of monomers or from preformed polymer with the possibility of performing many chemical modifications. According to the technologies used, nanospheres or nanocapsules can be obtained. Nanoparticle preparation methods based on the polymerization of monomers generally involve introducing the monomer to an aqueous phase or dissolving the monomer in a non-solvent of the polymer[17]. The polymerization reaction in these systems generally occurs in two steps: a nucleation phase followed by a growth phase. The process can be carried out in two ways either as emulsion polymerization or as interfacial polymerization. In emulsion polymerization, triggers for polymer growth are used such as high-energy radiation, UV light or hydroxyl ions. Emulsion polymerization offers many advantages: it is a fast process when compared to other processes; the process does not require stabilizers and surfactants; and the process can easily be scaled up. However, there are many challenges to the application of emulsion polymerization. These include (i) the requirement of organic solvents; (ii) the requirement for free-radical radiation or UV light used to trigger polymerization; this need for the triggers prevents the addition of proteins or peptides during polymerization. When nanoparticle preparation involves polymerization, it is undesirable to have residual monomers and initiators in the final nanoparticle formulation. A critical step of the process is the purification and removal of residual monomers. It is also very important to separate free (un-incorporated) drugs from the drug loaded nanoparticle suspension. Some of the methods of nanoparticle purification involving dialysis and centrifugation may be difficult to scale up in large manufacturing. The interfacial polymerization is similar to emulsion polymerization except that polymerization occurs when an aqueous and an organic phase are brought together by homogenization, emulsification or microfluidization under high-torque mechanical stirring. Drug incorporation is carried out by adding the drug with the monomer in the organic phase so as to ensure stability. A potential challenge for polymeric nanoparticles is associated with residues from organic solvents and polymer toxicity. In the polymer dispersion method, the polymer is dissolved in an organic solvent such as dichloromethane, chloroform or ethyl acetate. If the drug to be incorporated in nanoparticles is hydrophobic, the drug is dissolved in the polymer solution. The polymer solution is then added to an aqueous solution, followed by high-speed homogenization or sonication to form an oil-in-water emulsion. Nanoparticle preparation is usually facilitated and stabilized with the aid of an emulsifier or stabilizer. If the drug to be incorporated in nanoparticles is hydrophilic, the drug is added to the aqueous phase and entrapped into nanoparticles through a double emulsification method to form water-in-oil-in-water emulsion (double emulsification)[18]. Due to the implication on safety, it is important to remove organic solvent from the emulsion. Organic solvent can be removed by evaporation or a decreased pressure or under a vacuum environment with or without the aid of inert gas flow. Solid nanoparticles are cured from the suspension by centrifugation, filtration or freeze drying. Another method is based on particle precipitation upon addition of a non-solvent to polymer solution under mechanical stirring. This method allows the formation of nanoparticles without prior emulsification. Nanoparticle formation and characteristics are dependent on the choice of the polymer/solvent/non-solvent system that will ensure mutual miscibility of the solvent and non-solvent of the polymer. The method has been applied for many polymers like polylactide, polylactide-co-glycolide, polycaprolactone, ethycellulose, polyalkylcyanoacrylate and polystyrene. Nanoparticles can also be prepared from natural macromolecules using methods such as thermal denaturation of proteins (such as albumin) or gelification process such as in alginates. In general, the controlling factors in the nanoparticle formulation process, which are adjustable for an ideal design, are the polymer type and its molecular weight, the copolymer blend ratio, the type of organic solvent, the drug loading level, the emulsifier/stabilizer and oil–water phase ratio, the mechanical strength of mixing, the temperature and the pH. In the production of a drug product it is important to set a limit for residual solvent in the formulation that is based on the acceptable daily intake and to develop analytical methods for testing of the solvent levels in the nanoparticles[19] **(Figure 6.2)**

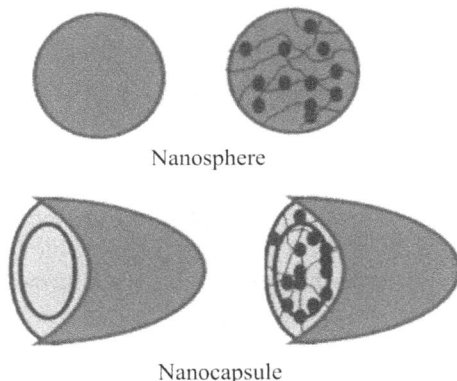

Nanosphere

Nanocapsule

Fig. 6.2 Polymeric nanoparticles.

(ii) Solid Lipid Nanoparticles

Solid lipid nanoparticles that are made from solid lipids using homogenization techniques and microemulsion methods[20]. Examples of lipids that are used include triglycerides (e.g., tristearin), partial glycerides (e.g., Imwitor), fatty acids (e.g., stearic acid), steroids (e.g., cholesterol) and waxes (e.g., cetyl palmitate). To prepare particles using the homogenization method, the drug is dissolved or solubilized in the lipid that has been melted and heated to a temperature approximately 5–108°C above its melting point. For the hot homogenization technique, the drug dissolved in the lipid melt is dispersed under stirring in a hot aqueous surfactant solution of identical temperature. The obtained pre-emulsion is homogenized to produce nanoemulsions that are subsequently cooled to room temperature. Solid lipid nanoparticles are obtained upon lipid recrystallization at room temperature **(Figure 6.3)**. Some of the process variables that will affect the particle size of nanoparticles as well as drug loading are (i) the type of homogenization technique; (ii) speed of homogenization; and (iii) rate of cooling in hot homogenization. Cold homogenization is applied for highly temperature-sensitive drugs and hydrophilic drugs. For the cold homogenization technique the drug containing lipid melt is cooled and ground to obtain lipid particles. The lipid particles are dispersed in a cold surfactant solution that is homogenized at or below room temperature. The process avoids or minimizes the melting of lipids and therefore minimizing the loss of hydrophilic drugs to the water surface. As mentioned previously, solid lipid nanoparticles can also be prepared by using microemulsions as precursors. Microemulsions are transparent, thermodynamically stable and easily manufactured systems. Essentially, microemulsions can be defined as small droplets (5–100 nm) of one liquid dispersed throughout another by virtue of the presence of fairly large concentrations of surfactants. Gasco reported SLN preparation techniques which are based on the dilution of microemulsions[21]. In this approach microemulsions are made by stirring an optically transparent mixture at 65–70 °C, which is composed of low-melting fatty acid (e.g., stearic acid), an emulsifier (e.g., polysorbate 20, polysorbate 60, soy phosphatidylcholine, taurodeoxycholic acid sodium salt), co-emulsifiers (e.g., butanol, sodium monooctylphosphate) and water. The hot microemulsion is dispersed in cold water (2–38 °C) under stirring using a typical volume ratio of the hot microemulsion to cold water in the range of 1:25–1:50. The dilution step is critically determined by the composition of the microemulsion. Other studies have investigated production of nanoparticles from warm microemulsions that required simple cooling of warm microemulsions at room temperature[22]. Microemulsions were prepared using materials such as waxes (e.g., emulsifying wax), polymeric surfactants such as Brij type, polyethylene glycol derivatives of fatty acids such as PEG-400 monostearate and phospholipids. The preparation of nanoparticles from microemulsion precursors is the platform technology that is being commercially applied to engineer drug and vaccine delivery systems (NaNoMed Pharmaceuticals; Kalamazoo, MI, USA). Important process factors in the application of microemulsions to prepare nanoparticles include (a) preparing a homogeneous mixture of lipids (or waxes) and drug; (b) achievement of substantial drug loading within microemulsion window; (c) cooling of the warm microemulsion to obtain nanoparticles; and (d) a purification process to remove excess surfactants and unincorporated drug from the nanoparticle suspension.

A commercial product that applies lipids in a nanoparticulate product is Doxil doxorubicin liposome (ALZA, Mountain View, CA, USA). Also, the lead product of Starpharma (Melbourne, Australia) is VivaGelTM which is a based on development of an anti-HIV drug through dendrimer nanotechnology. Using micellar nanoparticle technology, Novavax has developed an estrogen-containing product, Estrasorb (estradiol) that is approved by the US FDA.

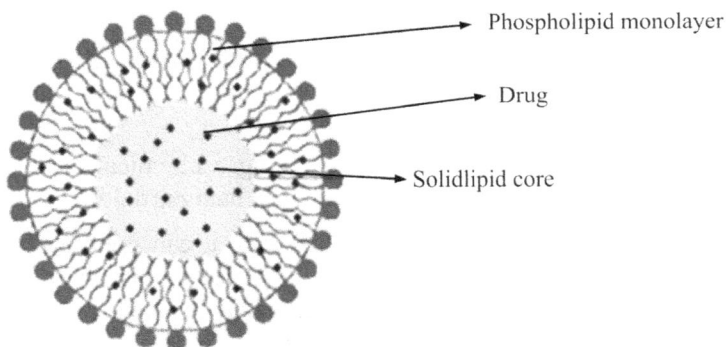

Fig. 6.3 Solid-lipid nanoparticle.

(iii) Nanoshells

A nanoshell is a type of spherical nanoparticle consisting of a dielectric core which is covered by a thin metallic shell (usually gold). These nanoshells involve a quasiparticle called plasmon which is a collective excitation or quantum plasma oscillation where the electrons simultaneously oscillate with respect to all the ions. The simultaneous oscillation can be called plasmon hybridization where the tunability of the oscillation is associated with mixture of the inner and outer shell where they hybridize to give a lower energy or higher energy. This lower energy couples strongly to incident light where as, the higher energy is an anti-bonding and weakly combines to incident light. The hybridization interaction is stronger for thinner shell layers; hence, the thickness of the shell and overall particle radius determines the wavelength of light. Nanoshells can be varied across a broad range of the light spectrum that spans the visible and near infrared regions. The interaction of light and nanoparticles affects the placements of charges which affects the coupling strength. Incident light polarized parallel to the substrate gives a s-polarization hence the charges are further from the substrate surface which gives a stronger interaction between the shell and core. Otherwise, a p-polarization is formed which gives a more strongly shifted plasmon energy causing a weaker interaction and coupling. A nanoshell is synthesized in a multistep process:

1. Obtain silica nanoparticles in a solution (usually tetrachloroauric acid and a reducing agent). There are several different reducing agents used and all can greatly affect the uniformity of the nanoparticle.

2. Attach a very small seed colloid onto the dielectric nanoparticles (such as: zinc selenide, sapphire, and glass) giving a discontinuous shell.

3. Grow a continuous shell by using a chemical reduction of the metal attached to the dielectric nanoparticles.

If a uniform shell is not obtained then it can greatly affect the optical properties of the nanoshell. A good example of this is a nanoegg, which is a metallic nanoshell that has a nonuniform thickness. This characteristic nonuniformity causes additional hybridized plasmon resonance in the spectrum making the coupling not as affective. Since nanoshells possess highly favorable optical and chemical properties it is often used for biomedical imaging, therapeutic applications, fluorescence enhancement of weak molecular emitters, surface enhanced Raman spectroscopy and surface enhanced infrared absorption spectroscopy. Gold nanoshells are shuttled into tumors by the use of phagocytosis where phagocytes engulf the nanoshells through the cell membrane to form an internal phagosome, or macrophage. After this it is shuttled into a cell and enzymes are usually used to metabolize it and shuttle it back out of the cell. These nanoshells are not metabolized so for them to be effective they just need to be within the tumor cells and photo induced cell death is used to terminate the tumor cells. This scheme is shown in **Figure 6.4.**

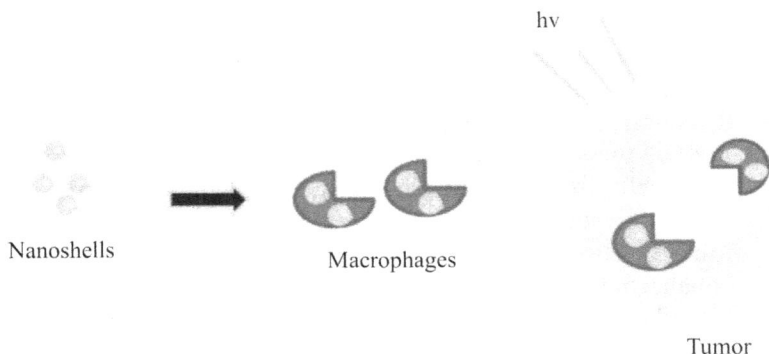

Fig. 6.4 Nanoshell tagetting to tumor cell.

Nanoparticle-based therapeutics have been successfully delivered into tumors by exploiting the enhanced permeability and retention effect, a property that permits nanoscale structures to be taken up passively into tumors with out the assistance of antibodies. Delivery of nanoshells into the important regions of tumors can be very difficult. This is where most nanoshells try to exploit the tumor's natural recruitment of monocytes for delivery as seen in the above figure. This delivery system is called a "Trojan Horse". This process works so well since tumors are about ¾ macrophages and once monocytes are brought into the tumor, it differentiates into macrophages which would also be need to maintain the cargo nanoparticles. Once the nanoshells are at the necrotic center, near-infrared illumination is used to destroy the tumor associated macrophages. Since nanoshells are easily optically tuned so that they absorb light in near infrared region, where there is a minimal optical absorption in tissue and penetration by the radiation is optimal for deep tissue treatments. Also prior to any illumination the nanoshell will be inert within the cell. Illumination is usually done by laser light, this light taken into nanoshell and converted into heat which increases the temperature of nanoshell to over 30 °C. This nanoshell-based photothermal ablation therapy shows success in mice with tumor remission with rates over 90%. The nanoshell's optical technologies give a high resolution and yet noninvasive functional imaging of tissues at a decent price. Unfortunately, the imaging is not very advanced since they have weak optical signals and subtle spectral differences of healthy and diseased tissue. There has been increasing interest in optical technologies with novel exogenous contrast agents, designed to define the molecular specific signatures of cancer, to improve the detection limits and clinical effectiveness of optical imaging. For a two dimensional hexagonal close-packed array of nanoshells with nanoscale gaps between nanoparticles, it enhances surface enhanced raman and surface enhanced infrared absorption signals. It is thought that the dominant enhancement mechanism is electromagnetic where the substrate provides the strong enhancements, superradiance. Superradiance is the coupling between adjacent resonant systems that results in an enhanced radiative damping. The field enhancements seen with mid-infrared resonance are caused by the "lightning-rod" effect. This effect occurs when metals are being efficient conductors and give off the electric field from the interior of the metals which channel the electric field into the junction between each nanoshell, resulting in large field intensities[23].

Polymeric Micelles

In the late 1960s, micelles drew much attention as drug carriers owing to their easily controlled properties and good pharmacological characteristics. Micelles are formed when amphiphiles are placed in water. They consist of an inner core of assembled hydrophobic segments capable of solubilizing lipophilic substances and an outer hydrophilic corona serving as a stabilizing interface between the hydrophobic core and the external aqueous environment. Depending on the delivery purpose, one can select the size, charge, and surface properties of these carriers simply by adding new ingredients to the mixture of amphiphilic substances before micelle preparation and/or by variation of the preparation method. Micelles as drug carriers provide a set of advantages—they physically entrap sparingly soluble pharmaceuticals and deliver them to the desired site of action at concentrations that can exceed their intrinsic water solubility, thus increase their bioavailability, stability of the drug and lessened undesirable side effects[24]. The most important feature of micellar delivery systems, which distinguish them from other particulate drug carriers, lies in their small size (~10 to 30 nm) and the narrow size distribution. Micelles made of nonionic surfactants are widely used as adjuvant and drug carrier systems in many areas of pharmaceutical technology and controlled drug delivery. Such a high level of activity has brought a great deal of diversity to this field, since most groups introduced their own micelle system formed from unique hydrophilic–hydrophobic combinations. In almost all cases, the hydrophilic outer shell consists of poly(ethylene oxide) (PEO) chains, owing to their high degree of hydration and large excluded volume inducing repulsive forces, which contribute to the stabilization of the micelle. In addition, the PEO corona prevents recognition by the reticuloendothelial system and therefore minimizes elimination of the micelle from the bloodstream. Thus, these so-called "stealth properties of the PEO corona result in increased blood circulation times and allow drugs to be administered over prolonged periods of time. A wide range of hydrophobic blocks have been explored, resulting in different micellar systems with distinct physicochemical properties. Surfactant micelles form only above a critical concentration, the critical micelle concentration (CMC), and rapidly break apart upon dilution, which can result in premature leakage of the drug and its precipitation in situ. These limitations of surfactant micelles as drug delivery carriers triggered the search for micelles of significantly enhanced stability and solubilizing power. The use of polymer-based micelles has gained much attention because of the high diversity of polymers, their biocompatibility, biodegradibility, and the multiplicity of functional groups they display for the conjugation of pilot molecules **(Figure 6.5).**

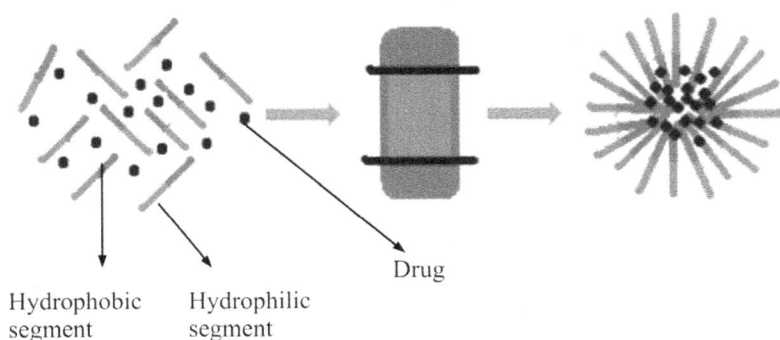

Drug

Hydrophobic segment   Hydrophilic segment

Fig. 6.5 Formation of Nanoshell.

5. Dendrimers

Dendrimers are a newer class of polymeric drug delivery devices with a unique macromolecular structure. The three-dimensional complexes are produced in an iterative sequence of reaction steps leading to generations of branches organized around an inner core. The hierarchical synthesis of these complexes lends itself to finely controlled size, composition, and reactivity. Poly(amidoamine) dendrimers were the first constructed and characterized, but dozens of other dendrimer types have been investigated to date[25]. Dendrimers are formed either by divergent or convergent methods, each having its own advantages and disadvantages. The behavior and characteristics of dendrimers can differ greatly from their linear counterparts. Due to their step-wise synthesis, the polydispersity of dendrimers is quite low, contributing to their utility as drug delivery devices. The scaffold provides an ideal platform for drug molecules that does not depend on thermodynamics or physical factors. The choice of polymer used in the dendritic system plays heavily into its utility as a drug carrier owing to the association between the polymer and drug molecule. The drug indomethacin was loaded (11 wt%) into dendritic micelles composed of a hydrophobic Fre´chet-type dendrimer and a shell of hydrophilic poly(ethylene glycol) by Fre´chet et al. The release of the drug from the complex was much slower than that of the same drug from a cellulose membrane, all drug was released over 25 hours as opposed to 4 hours with the cellulose. 5-Fluorouracil has been incorporated into poly (amidoamine) dendrimers augmented with PEG-500. The complexation between the hydrophilic drug and dendrimer occurred with incubation. *In vitro* release from the PEGylated dendrimers occurred over 6 days, whereas the non-PEGylated formulations released all drug over 1 day (Bhadra, Bhadra et al. 2003). For entrapment within the dendrimer, drugs may be electrostatically or covalently bound to the surface of the dendrime (**Figure 6.6**).

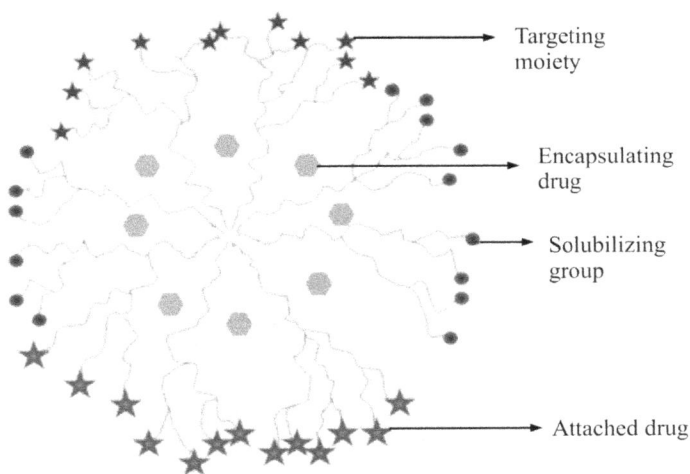

Fig. 6.6 Dendrimers.

6. Viral Vectors

Viral vectors have been proposed as efficient gene delivery devices due to their evolutionary advantage over man-made colloidal systems for transfection of cells. Synthetic or modified viruses carry the therapeutic gene in their capsid, being able to protect it until it reaches its intended target. Many exciting strides have been made in this field, yet many hurdles remain to make the device safe and viable *in vivo*[26]. Various examples are classes of nanoscale-controlled delivery devices exist including protein-based delivery devices, magnetic nanoparticles, inorganic nanoparticles, and others.

7. Nanocrystals

Fahlman, B. D. has described a nanocrystal as any nanomaterial with at least one dimension ≤ 100 nm and that is single crystalline. More properly, any material with a dimension of less than 1 micrometre, i.e., 1000 nanometers, should be referred to as a nanoparticle, not a nanocrystal. For example, any particle which exhibits regions of crystallinity should be termed nanoparticle or nanocluster based on dimensions. Crystalline nanoparticles are of interest because they often provide single-domain crystalline systems that can be studied to provide information that can help explain the behaviour of macroscopic samples of similar materials, without the complicating presence of grain boundaries and other defects. Crystalline nanoparticles made with zeolite are used as a filter to turn crude oil onto diesel fuel at an ExxonMobil oil refinery in Louisiana, a method cheaper than the conventional way. A layer of crystalline nanoparticles is used in a new type of solar panel named Solar Ply made by Nanosolar. It is cheaper than other solar panels, more flexible, and claims 12% efficiency. (Conventionally inexpensive organic solar panels convert 9% of the sun's energy into electricity.) Crystal tetrapods 40 nanometers wide convert photons into electricity, but only have 3% efficiency. The term NanoCrystal is a registered trademark of Elan Pharma International Limited (Ireland) used in relation to Elan's proprietary milling process and nanoparticulate drug formulations. Rapamune was previously available only as an oral solution in bottles or sachets - requires refrigeration storage and must be mixed with water/orange juice prior to administration[27]. The new tablet developed with Nanocrystal technology having particle size less than 200nm and coating the active compound with surface stabilizers provides patients with more convenient administration and storage. The nanocrystals provides the greater surface which is illustrated in **Figure 6.7**.

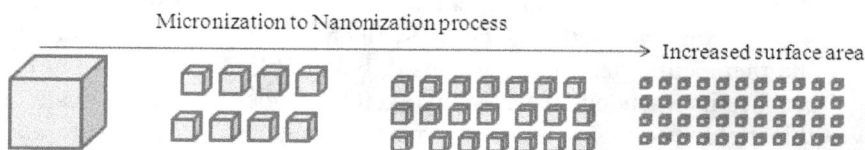

Fig. 6.7 Nanocrystals.

Nanotubes, Nanorods, Nanofibers, and Fullerenes

Nanotubes

Carbon nanotubes (CNT) have shown substantial potential in a variety of biological applications including use as DNA and protein biosensors, ion channel blockers, bioseparators and biocatalysts[28]. This potential stems from their specific surface or adaptable size-dependent properties in combination with their anisotropic character. Their anisotropy is of consequence since it influences their electronic, photonic, mechanical, and chemical properties[29]. The first successful multi-walled carbon nanotube synthesis was demonstrated in 1991, and the first single-walled carbon nanotube synthesis followed in 1993[30]. Multiple methods of synthesis have subsequently been reported. These include self assembly of precursor compounds[31], vapor deposition[32], and template synthesis[33]. The method of synthesis determines its innate physicochemical properties.

Carbon nanotubes are cylindrical macromolecules with variable radii starting at a few nanometers with maximum lengths up to 20 cm. CNTs have an allotropic crystalline carbonic form that is consistent with fullerenes[34]. There are two main types of carbon nanotubes, single-wall carbon nanotube (SWCNT), which is composed of a hexagonal lattice of carbon atoms equivalent to atomic planes of graphite ranging in diameter from 7 to 16 A$^{o[35]}$. The second is the multi-wall carbon nanotube (MWCNT), consisting of a concentric arrangement of similar graphene sheets that are spaced by a distance of approximately 3.4 A$^{o[36]}$. These MWCNTs can reach diameters of up to 100 nm (Lu 1997). Both single- and multi-walled tubes are capped at their ends by one half of a fullerene-like molecule[37]. However, open-ended tubules have also been reported[38]. In addition, nanotubes are able, due to strong Vander Waals forces, to self-organize into hexagonal-ordered rope-like structures consisting of 50–100 tubes that range in lengths up to several microns[39]. Carbon nanotubes are generally acknowledged as the ultimate carbon fiber with a high strength and superior thermal conductivity. A CNT can behave as a metal or a semiconductor, depending on its chiral vector[40]. According to molecular dynamics simulations, CNTs have a Young's modulus several times greater than that of diamond[41] and also possess enhanced field emission properties. The chemical modification and solubilization of carbon nanotubes is essential to their successful application in drug delivery. In addition, nanotubes have the advantage of facile DNA, peptide, or other molecular incorporation into their hollow space[42]. Ideal SWCNTs contain two separate regions, each with a unique reactivity toward covalent chemical modification. The intermittent five-membered rings on the caps increase reactivity at these points to levels similar to fullerenes. The functionalization of carbon nanotubes can broadly be divided into two categories: (a) direct attachment of functional groups to the graphitic surface and (b) the use of the nanotube-bound carboxylic acids[43]. For example, functionalization of CNTs using polyethylene-oxide chains has been achieved by using carboxylic acid end groups[44]. This imparts the nanotubes with enhanced water solubility and non-specific protein-resistant properties. Surface functionalization in this manner enables adsorption or attachment of various molecules or antigens. This provides a mechanism for specific recognition and cell targeting[45]. Nanotubes, therefore, have significant potential for targeted drug delivery.

Nanotubes have displayed low toxicity but this is dependent on the route of administration and surface functionalization. The high aspect ratio of carbon nanotubes gives them unique toxicological profiles[46]. For example, exposure of human epidermal keratinocytes (HaCaT) to unrefined and unfunctionalized SWCNT has been shown to result in increased oxidative stress resulting in accelerated free radical generation, accumulation of peroxidative products, a decrease of intracellular levels of glutathione, oxidation of protein SH groups, and depletion of total antioxidant reserve and vitamin E 18 hours after exposure. Ultrastructure and morphological changes were also observed in the cells[47]. Cellular toxicity has been attributed to the insolubility of non-functionalized carbon nanotubes and the associated traces of catalyst materials such as nickel, iron, or cobalt. To overcome this, nanotubes can be purified via oxidation with strong acid treatments that allow for the removal of the metallic impurities. Moreover, it has been shown that peptide-functionalized CNTs are able to enhance an antibody-mediated response against the peptide with no discernable cross-reactivity to the nanotubes themselves, thus demonstrating a lack of immunogenicity[48].

Carbon nanotubes enhance uptake of small molecules, large proteins, and amino acids that have previously demonstrated low cellular penetration. This cell-penetrating ability can be enhanced further by conjugation of cell-penetrating peptides onto the carbon nanotubes.

Because carbon nanotubes have a high loading capacity for cargo molecules due to their innately high aspect ratios, they have the potential to be ideal shuttles for peptide antigens. Carbon nanotubes with attached protein conjugates have been found to possess antibody recognition equal to that of free peptides, indicating that the integrity and functionality of a nanotube-linked peptide is maintained. The mechanism for cellular uptake of nanotubes is not yet entirely understood. However, two routes of internalization have been proposed. In the first, functionalized nanotubes have been shown to penetrate a cell via passive diffusion across the lipid bilayer in a needle-like manner. The second mechanism stems from the observation that cellular endocytosis serves as the route for internalization of CNTs with adsorbed surface proteins.

Nanorods

Nanorods have unique innate chemical, electrical, magnetic, and optical anisotropy, thus allowing them to interact with cells, tissues, and biomolecules in fundamentally novel ways[49]. The two most frequently used methods of manufacturing nanorods involve template. Template synthesis involves electrochemical deposition into a non-conducting membrane that has an array of cylindrical pores[50]. Subsequent removal of the membrane by etching yields metallic nanorods of controlled dimensions. Template synthesis is advantageous because it is easily adapted for the deposition of multiple submicrometer segments produce large quantities of monodisperse nanorods, and properties such as aspect ratio can be controlled in a systematic way (Salem et al. 2003). Metallic nanorods for bio applications are most frequently synthesized from gold, copper, platinum, or silver[51]. Inorganic metallic nanorods are obtainable on a micron to A° scale[52], and possess physical and chemical characteristics completely unique of their bulk properties. Gold is the most widely used inorganic material in diagnostic and delivery nanoparticulate research. Gold nano properties are different from bulk properties because of a change in the quantum confinement of electron motion[53]. As particles become smaller, their surface: interior atomic ratio increases until the surface properties become a primary behavioral factor. Gold nanoparticles have been used to demonstrate multiphoton absorption-induced luminescence (MAIL), where particular tissues or cells are fluorescently labeled. Gold nanoparticles emit light that is so intense easily possible to observe a single nanoparticle at laser intensities lower than those commonly used for MAIL. Gold nanorods allow for a simple bottom-up approach to the development of nanoscale delivery systems. In comparison to spherical particles, asymmetric particles offer additional degrees of freedom in self-assembly due to their inherent shape anisotropy[54].

This ability to engineer nanorods with multiple functionalities in spatially defined regions offers the potential for increased efficacy for drug and gene delivery systems over alternative single-component inorganic non-viral vectors[55]. For example, we have assembled a non-viral gene delivery system based on multi segment bimetallic nanorods that can simultaneously bind compacted DNA plasmids and targeting ligands in a spatially defined manner. The physicochemical properties of nanorods are major factors in the characteristic biodistribution and residence times of these particles *in vivo*[56]. For example, particle size is a significant determinant of extravasation rate, and surface charge can impact non-specific uptake and degradation by macrophages. Additionally, particles with engineered hydrophobic surfaces are preferentially taken up by the liver, followed by the spleen and lungs[57]. Similar to nanotubes, nanorods offer significant potential in the formation of cell-penetrating complexes for drug or probe molecule delivery.

Nanofibers

In the areas of tissue engineering and drug delivery, nanofibers have emerged as biocompatible, biodegradable scaffolds, and delivery vehicles. They are used for the replacement of tissues with structural or physiological deficiencies. The use of nanofibers in tissue restoration can potentially produce an efficient, compact organ with a rapid recovery process. This is because of the large surface area that polymer and protein-based nanofibers possess. The large surface area helps to support cell growth on the scaffold materials, wound healing, the construction of biocompatible prostheses and bone substitutes, implant epithelialization, and drug delivery applications. Nanofibrous scaffolds designed to elicit specific cellular responses through the incorporation of signaling ligands, such as growth factors or DNA fragments, show particular promise for future treatment strategies[58]. Nanofibers of different chemistries and structures can be formed by self-assembly at the molecular level. These nanofibers have potential applications in the promotion of cell adhesion and growth, targeted drug delivery, tissue engineering, and filtration systems for toxic chemicals[59]. For example, the pentapeptide epitope IKVAV is an amino acid sequence of laminin that promotes neurite adhesion. Amphiphiles that present this sequence can self-assemble in aqueous media, or at the site of injection in tissues, and fibers with a diameter of 5–10 nm are formed[60]. These scaffolds discourage astrocyte development while inducing prompt differentiation to neurons. These findings suggest that synthetic materials such as these self-assembling nanofibers may have the ability to modulate selective gene expression. The nanofibers contain multiple binding sites for heparin and other compounds necessary for new blood vessel growth. The release of these proteins as nanofibers break down can stimulate neighboring cells for continued growth[61]. An alternative approach to natural collagen is the use of synthetic collagen substitutes that self assemble into nanocylindrical structures. The nanofiber is made up of a long hydrophobic alkyl group on one end and a hydrophilic peptide on the other end. These nanocylinders can direct the formation of hydroxyl apatite crystallites with dimensions and orientations similar to those in natural bone. Therefore, self-assembled nanofibers have unique properties with significant potential for drug delivery applications.

The potential for nanofiber production for use in tissue engineering and as filters for toxic chemicals has generated increased interest in the electrospinning process. Nanofibers can be created from synthetic polymers, such as polylactides or polyamides, as well as natural polymers, such as collagen, silk, and celluloses. The polymers are spun into nanofibers using organic solvents like chloroform, ethanol, or formic acid, and water is used in the spinning solution. The spinning parameters of solution concentration, viscosity, electrical conductivity, surface free energy, and solvent permeability affect the diameter of the nanofibers and their resulting surface topology, which may be smooth or porous. Nanofibers may be produced with diameters ranging from a few nanometers to a few micrometers. However, the length can theoretically be infinitely long[62]. Self-assembled nanofibers will align themselves into distinctive 3D patterns such as honeycomb meshes on a collector substrate. These "nanowebs" give increased trapping and filtering mechanisms that have potential for use in chemical defense masks and protective clothing. Additionally, the polymer nanofiber based filtration devices are now commercially developed for industrial air filtrations, as filters for gas turbine generators and filters for heavy duty engines. Besides offering an opportunity to generate ultra-thin diameters, small size porosity, and suitable surface morphology, the electrospinning process can provide fiber carriers for drug delivery with attractive features on multiple levels. For example, drugs can be conveniently incorporated into the carrier polymers without structural and bioactive alteration. The small diameter of the nanofibers can provide a short diffusion passage length, and the high surface area facilitates mass transfer and efficient drug release[63].

For effective cell interactions, polymer nanofibers often need to be functionalized to yield increased bioactivity and fiber–cell interaction properties. The addition of other molecules such as genes, drugs, growth factors, and other ligands directly to the polymer solution or melt prior to electrospinning will produce functionalized, bioactive nanofibers. For example, plasmid DNA has been added directly to solutions of PLA–PEG and PLGA in dimethylformamide (DMF) prior to electrospinning for nanofiber production. Surface modification can also be used to functionalize polymeric nanofibers. With degradable polymer nanofibers, special care must be taken to protect the nanofibers from rapid degradation and destruction. Strong reaction conditions such as exposure to plasma, ultraviolet, or gammaradiation, high temperatures, and acidic or basic environments can easily degrade the nanofibers. Additionally, the high surface area of biodegradable nanofibers such as PLA and PGA tends to degrade much faster compared with bulk materials. Polyethylene terephthalate (PET) nanofibers showed significant degradation in acidic or basic solutions[64].

Polymer nanofibers have shown good compatibility with other tissues when used as scaffolds and matrices. Fibers made of natural materials show the most promising compatibility. When human bone marrow stromal cells are grown on fibroin-based nanofibers, these electrospun silk matrices are able to support cell attachment and growth in culture over a 2-week period[65]. Human keratinocytes and fibroblasts have also been reported to attach and proliferate on these fibroin-based nanofibers.

Fullerenes

Fullerenes are a recently discovered class of carbon allotropes, found in hollow spherical ellipse or tube shapes. The entire class of these closed caged carbon molecules is called fullerenes. The C60 fullerene is commonly referred to as a buck ball, in honor of Buckminster Fuller[66]. Fullerenes have potential applications in the treatment of diseases where oxidative stress plays a role in the pathogenesis, such as neurodegenerative diseases. Another possible application of fullerenes is in nuclear medicine, as an alternative to chelating compounds that prevent the direct binding of toxic metal ions to serum components. This could increase the therapeutic potency of radiation treatments and decrease their adverse effects because fullerenes are resistant to biochemical degradation within the body. The hydrophobic C60 molecule can be modified to include covalently bonded hydrophilic molecules, which increase the solubility and potential use in biological applications. Water-soluble fullerenes are able to cross the cell membrane[67]. Metallofullerenes are all-carbon fullerenes that enclose metal ions to deliver radioactive atoms directly to diseased tissues, such as cancer. This has the potential to decrease the side effects of non-targeted radiation treatments, since the radioactive atoms will not damage healthy surrounding tissue. This is one example of the potential drug delivery applications of the fullerene family[68].

Within the past 10 years, the physical and chemical properties of fullerenes have gained increasing interest as scientists try to understand how these properties can be exploited to yield new treatments and applications. Fullerenes can be produced through combustion and oxidation of benzene and argon gas mixtures, by resistive heating of carbon rods in vacuum, or through laser vaporization. The most commonly used and most efficient method involves running a large current between two nearby graphite electrodes in an inert atmosphere, such as helium, at a pressure of 200 Torr. A carbon plasma arc will be formed between the electrodes, and the cooled carbon soot contains fullerenes that must be extracted and then purified.

Fullerene-binding molecules have potential in drug delivery applications. For example, they could facilitate specific antibiotics targeting resistant bacteria or drugs targeting cancer cells such as melanoma. Other examples include the use of fullerenes as light-activated antimicrobial agents[69]. Fullerenes are the only known carbon allotrope that can be dissolved in common solvents at room temperature, and are moderately soluble in nonpolar and weakly polar solvents. At the same time, the fact that they are nanosized means that they can be treated as colloidal particles. This is observed when the solid phase of fullerenes is added to a liquid, and a molecular solution is first formed. Subsequently, dispersion forces will cause the fullerenes to cluster into a colloidal solution[70]. While no single parameter can be used to predict the solubility of a fullerene in a solvent, several general trends have been found to govern their behavior in a particular solvent. The solubility in a solvent generally increases with increasing molecular weight of the solvent. An increase in the polarizability parameter generates higher solubilities. The solubility of a selected solvent will be important in its successful use in the further extraction and purification of fullerenes. On their own, fullerenes are not readily soluble in water, so a solubilization method is necessary for the fullerene acting in biological systems. A fairly quick method involves solubilization by tetrahydrofuran (THF), mixing with water, and then evaporation to eliminate the THF. The water stirred method is simply weeks of water stirring. This method is more environmentally friendly than the previous method, but takes a considerable amount of time. However, studies have shown that fullerenes produced by the THF method exhibit higher toxicities in vivo, possible because of residual solvent trapped within the fullerene.

Because fullerenes have numerous points of attachment, they have the ability to give control to the 3D positioning of chemical groups onto their structure. This improves their ability to target specific cells and molecules. The 60 carbons in the buckyball formation, for example, give 60 points of attachment for forming a more complex delivery assembly[71]. This, along with their nanosize dimensions, redox potential, and ability to encapsulate other molecules, makes fullerenes an attractive candidate for drug delivery applications. Water-soluble derivatives of C60 fullerenes have shown uptake and localization primarily in the mitochondria. Additionally, researchers have found that fullerenes react with damaging oxygen free radicals through their C–C double bonds. This binding occurs so quickly that only diffusion controls the reaction. This means that the fullerene will bind the radical each time it encounters one. By binding and inactivating these free radicals that circulate throughout the body, fullerenes could be used to treat diseases caused by excessive free radical production. Fullerene antioxidants could provide more effective therapies for CNS-degenerative diseases such as Parkinson's disease, which is currently only marginally treated by natural and synthetic antioxidants[72]. Fullerenes have also demonstrated antiprotease activity which has the potential for use in treatment of human immunodeficiency virus and acquired immunodeficiency syndrome. There is conflicting evidence on whether fullerenes are relatively inert or potentially harmful to the body. When fullerenes were dispersed in water at concentrations of 0.5 parts per million and evaluated in largemouth bass, it was found that the fish suffered a 17-fold increase in cellular damage in the brain tissue after 48 hours. Fullerenes induced lipid peroxidation, which has been shown to impair the functioning of cell membranes and lead to cellular damage. Inflammatory changes also occurred in the liver and genes that are related to the making of repair enzymes. The damage to lipid-rich tissues likely occurred because the fullerenes are redox active. To overcome this limitation further research into biocompatible coatings that eliminate the redox-reactive surface while still allowing for drug delivery is necessary **(Figure 6.8).**

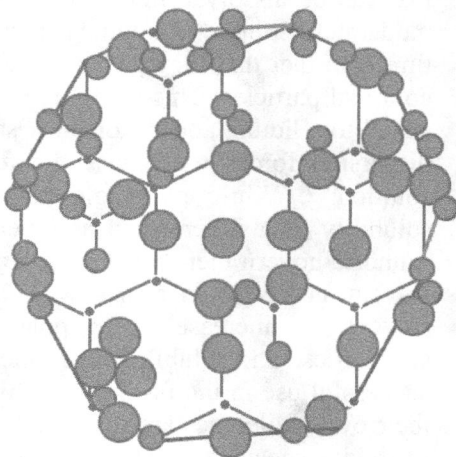

Fig. 6.8 Fullerenes.

Advances in Drug Delivery Systems based on Nanotechnology

1. Smart Drug Delivery Systems

Nanotechnology has a great impact on the development of polymeric drug delivery systems. One of the most outstanding achievements in the drug delivery field is the development of smart drug delivery systems (SDDSs), also called stimuli-sensitive delivery systems. The concept of SDDS is based on rapid transitions of a physicochemical property of polymer systems upon an environmental stimulus, which includes physical (temperature, mechanical stress, ultrasound, electricity, light), chemical (pH, ionic strength), or biological (enzymes, biomolecules) signals. Such stimuli can be either "internal" signals, resulting from changes in the physiological condition of a living subject, or "external" signals, artificially induced to provoke desired events. SDDS provides a programmable and predictable drug release profile in response to various stimulation sources. Depending on the applications, one can design on–off system, pulsatile/sustained drug release, and closed-loop drug delivery systems, for enhanced therapeutic efficiency with low systemic toxicity and side effects. SDDS provides various advantages over conventional drug delivery systems **(Figure 6.9).** The conventional controlled release systems are based on the predetermined drug release rate irrespective of the environmental condition at the time of application. On the other hand, SDDS is based on the release-on-demand strategy, allowing a drug carrier to liberate a therapeutic drug only when it is required in response to a specific stimulation. The best example of SDDS has been self-regulated insulin delivery systems that can respond to changes in the environmental glucose level[73-74]. One of the most widely used SDDSs has been polymeric micelles. Many polymeric micelles consisting of hydrophobic and hydrophilic polymer blocks have been developed. They can dissolve water-insoluble drugs, such as doxorubicin or paclitaxel, at high concentrations. When polymeric micelles are administered to the body, usually into the blood stream, drug release from polymeric micelles depends on simple diffusion, degradation of the micelle blocks, or disruption of the micelles by body components. Although release kinetics of the loaded drug can be modulated by varying the degradation rate of hydrophobic polymer blocks, the degradation rate is usually very slow, and thus, the loaded drug is released by diffusion from polymeric micelles. This slow release by passive diffusion may not be desirable, as the polymeric micelles reaching the target site need to release their contents fast. To alleviate this problem, smart polymeric micelles have been designed to liberate the loaded therapeutic agent at the targeted site fast. Poly(ethylene glycol)-b-polyhistidine (PEG-b-PHis), for instance, forms micelles only over the pKb of the PHis block (pH 6.5–7.0)[75]. The pKb can be adjusted by varying the molecular weight of PHis. Since solid tumors have a slightly acidic environment, a small reduction in pH to less than 7 at the tumor site triggers dissociation of the polymeric micelle to dump its contents. PEG-b-PHis micelles containing doxorubicin effectively killed multi-drug resistant (MDR) MCF-7 cells at pH 6.8[76]. The SDDS can achieve a highly localized drug accumulation at the target site[77] even though it is administered by systemic injection. The SDDS with enhanced targeting capability is highly promising in increasing the efficiency and efficacy of therapy with minimal side effects.

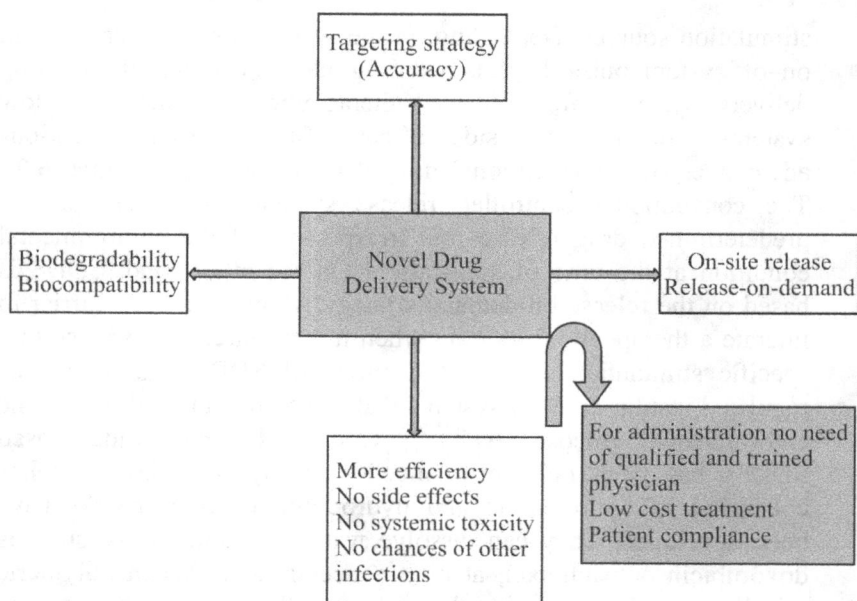

Fig. 6.9 Advantages of SDDs.

2. Polymer–Drug Conjugates

The polymer–drug conjugate itself can be considered as a nanovehicle. Various conjugates have been developed and clinically tested since the first drug conjugate for cancer therapy was proposed in the middle of 1970 s[78]. Recent advances in polymer–drug conjugates are well described in excellent reviews[79]. One of the major advantages of polymer–drug conjugates is prolonged circulation in the blood stream by retarding degradation/ metabolism/ excretion rates of the conjugated drugs. Many peptide and protein drugs cannot be delivered by oral administration because of their large molecular weights. Even when administered directly into the blood stream, they do not remain in the blood for a long time due to fast degradation and metabolism, limiting the clinical applications. The circulation times of these drugs have increased substantially by conjugation with polymers, such as PEG. For example, PEGylated form of Lasparaginase increased the plasma half-life up to 357 h, which was about 15 times longer than the natural form of L-asparaginase (half-life 20 h)[80]. The PEG-L-asparaginase received an FDA approval for clinical use. Another example is glucagon-like peptide-1 (GLP-1) which regulates food uptake and insulin release. GLP-1 is a very useful therapeutic agent for diabetic patients, but it is liable to degradation by a plasma enzyme, dipeptidyl dipeptidase IV. By introducing one PEG chain, its half-life was increased up to 40 folds over a natural form. The polymer conjugation, especially PEGylation[81] appears to be a useful technology for developing new polymer–drug conjugates. Another attractive feature of polymer–drug conjugates is the biodegradable linkage between the polymer backbone and the conjugated drug molecules. One well-known example is based on N-(2-hydroxypropyl)-methacrylamide (HPMA)[82-84]. Although 584 S. Kim *et al.* the backbone polymer is not degradable, therapeutic drugs are suspended to the backbone via a degradable linkage. Once the conjugate enters into cells, the linkage is readily hydrolyzed by lysosomal enzymes[85]. Usually, drugs with low molecular weight and high hydrophobicity have been used for conjugation. The degradation/ clearance rate and toxicity of a conjugated drug, i.e., prodrug, are greatly reduced, and the therapeutic effect is achieved only by hydrolysis inside the target cells to release the original drug. The polymers used in conjugation can have stimuli-responsiveness, providing a unique property to the conjugated drug. The activity of a conjugated drug can be turned on or off by external signals. For example, endoglucanase 12A (EG 12A), which had one site mutation (N55C) near the active site, was conjugated with either photo-sensitive[86] or thermo-sensitive polymers[87]. As a result, the catalytic activity of EG 12A could be turned on by application of UV light or high temperature. The active site of the enzyme was exposed by collapsing the conjugated long polymer chain by external stimuli. Once visible light was turned on or the temperature was lowered, the enzyme activity vanished due to the blocking of the active site by the extended polymer chain.

3. Multifunctional Drug Carriers

A multifunctional drug delivery system (MDDS) has two or more functions. SDDS and polymer–drug conjugates can be considered MDDS, because, in addition to delivering drugs, they can carry out the second function, such as stimuli-responsiveness or hydrolysis inside cells. Delivering drugs, however, should be considered as the inherent property for drug delivery systems, and thus, the MDDS is limited to the drug carrier that has multiple properties of prolonged blood circulation, passive or active localization at specific disease site, stimuli-sensitivity, ability to deliver drug into intracellular target organelles, and/or imaging ability[88]. The goal of MDDS is to maximize the therapeutic efficiency of a drug loaded in nanocarriers as well as to minimize undesirable side effects of the drug. A good example of MDDS is biotin-tagged pH-sensitive polymeric micelles based on a mixture of PLA-b-PEG-b-PHis-biotin (PLA= poly (L-lactic acid)) and PEG-b-PHis block copolymers. In that system, even the targeting moiety, biotin, was masked until the carrier was exposed to an expected environment of pH 7.0. Once the nanocarrier was internalized to cancer cells by ligand–receptor interactions, lowered pH (< 6.5) destabilized the carrier resulting in a burst release of the loaded drug. A more complicated example is a pH-degradable PEG-b-phosphatidylethanolamine (PE) liposome with attached anti-myosin monoclonal antibody as well as TAT or biotin on its surface[89-90]. The liposome integrated pH sensitivity and double-targeting moieties in a single particle.

4. Organic/Inorganic Composites

Recently, a series of review papers on the lab-on-a-chip (LOC) approach was published[91-95]. The LOC is a micro/nano-electro-mechanical system (MEMS/NEMS) which embodies micron- or nano-sized machines composed of sophisticated circuits. Such microfluidic systems can miniaturize huge instruments, e.g., GPC, HPLC, and electrophoresis systems, into a single chip. Small devices provide many advantages including portability/disposability, low cost, high reproducibility, high-throughput screening, and multiple functionalities in a single device. In addition, combined with other technologies such as optics, single molecular imaging, or cell/protein-based assay systems, the BioMEMS or BioNEMS of biomedical LOC devices become an important part of drug discovery and diagnosis. Drug delivery systems based on MEMS/NEMS are just beginning to appear[96-97]. To release a drug from a nanodevice is more complicated than to perform assay or screening drug candidates. Successful drug delivery requires at least four components: drug reservoir, pump, valve, and sensor[98]. Drugs can be placed either in a fabricated reservoir of a MEMS/NEMS device or in conventional micro-/ nanoparticles. Depending on the characteristics of a drug or a disease, different kinds of pumps (e.g., pulsatile, osmotic, or actuating) can be used. Since the valve and sensor directly contact biological constituents, good biocompatibility is essential. By adopting smart polymers as valves and sensors, versatility in drug release control can be obtained[99]. One of the problems with MEMS/NEMS-based drug delivery systems is that the operating protocol is not user-friendly. Due to the complicated and highly integrated structure, operation is limited to highly trained people, although such devices have been originally designed for general users without professional skills. BioMEMS/BioNEMS systems still remain in the research domain, and more improvement is necessary for developing clinically useful systems.

Other important organic/inorganic composites are metal nano-particles, such as quantum dot, iron oxide, or gold nanoparticles, coated with hydrophilic polymers. Their major application has been in diagnostic applications. Semi-conductive quantum dots emit sharp visible/near infrared lights with a wide range of wavelength by tuning the particle size (5–20 nm). Due to their high photostability, many quantum dots have been studied for optical diagnostic imaging of diseases as well as for labeling biomolecules. The critical problem with quantum dot applications is their inherent toxicity, because quantum dots are composed of heavy metals. Gold nanoparticles that emit red light around 520 nm have also been used for drug delivery and bioimaging[100]. Recently, gold nanoshell was developed, which provided tunable emission light for bioimaging[101]. In addition, gold nanoparticles can be detected by X-ray and emit thermal energy by excitation. For this reason, nano-sized gold particles are useful for medical imaging and thermal therapy. Super paramagnetic iron oxide (SPIO) nanoparticles have been developed for magnetic resonance imaging (MRI) of the whole body[102]. These nanoparticles are primarily engulfed by monocyte or macrophage after intravenous administration.However, uptake of SPIO by macrophage does not induce activation of nearby cells. This is why SPIO nanoparticles can be used for diagnosis of inflammatory or degenerative diseases. By introducing homing markers, spatial resolution of MRI can be improved significantly.

In-situ gelling system: Ideally, an *insitu* gelling system should be a low viscous, free flowing liquid to allow for reproducible administration to the eye as drops, and the gel formed following phase transition should be strong enough to with stand the shear forces in the *culdesac* and demonstrated long residence times in the eye. In order to increase the effectiveness of the drug a dosage form should be chosen which increases the contact time of the drug in the eye. This may then prolonged residence time of the gel formed *in situ* along with its ability to release drugs in sustained manner will assist in enhancing the bioavailability, reduce systemic absorption and reduce the need for frequent administration leading to improved patient compliance[103]. Depending upon the method employed to cause sol to gel phase transition on the ocular surface, the following types of systems are recognized:

- pH-triggered systems: cellulose acetate phthalate(CAP) latex, carbopol, polymethacrilic acid(PMMA), polyethylene glycol (PEG), pseudolatexes.

- Temperature dependent systems: chitosan, pluronics, tetronics, xyloglucans, hydroxypropylmethyl cellulose or hypromellose (HPMC).

- Ion-activated systems (osmotically induced gelation): gelrite, gellan, hyaluronic acid, alginates.

- UV induced gelation

- Solvent exchange induced gelation.

These (liquid) vehicles undergo a viscosity increase upon instillation in the eye, thus favouring precorneal retention. Such a change in viscosity can be triggered mainly by a change in temperature, pH or electrolyte composition.

pH triggered *in situ* gelation: Polyacrylic acid (Carbopol 940) is used as the gelling agent in combination with hydroxypropyl-methylcellulose (Methocel E50LV) which acted as a viscosity enhancing agent. The formulation with pH-triggered *in situ* gel is therapeutically efficacious, stable, non-irritant and provided sustained release of the drug for longer period of time than conventional eye drops. Another example cellulose acetate phthalate (CAP) is a polymer undergoing coagulation when the original pH of the solution (4.5) is raised to 7.4 by the tear fluid[104-106].

Temperature triggered *in situ* gel: The system is designed to use Poloxamer as a vehicle for ophthalmic drug delivery using *in situ* gel formation property. The gelation temperature of graft copolymers can be determined by measuring the temperature at which immobility of the meniscus in each solution was first noted. The bioadhesive and thermally gelling of these graft copolymers expected to be an excellent drug carrier for the prolonged delivery to surface of the eye. Other example Poloxamer-407 (a polyoxyethylenepolyoxypropylene block copolymer, Pluronic F-127® is a polymer with a solution viscosity that increases when its temperature is raised to the eye temperature[107-108].

Ionactivated *in situ* gelation: Alginate (Kelton) is used as the gelling agent in combination with HPMC (Methocel E50Lv) which acted as a viscosity-enhancing agent. Gelrite gellan gum, a novel ophthalmic vehicle that gels in the presence of mono or divalent cations, present in the lachrymal fluid can be used alone and in combinations with sodium alginate as the gelling agent[109-110].

Solid Dosage Forms

Films, erodible and non-erodible inserts, rods and shields are the most logical delivery systems aimed at remaining for a long period of time in the front of the eye. These delivery systems sustain and control drug release and thus avoid pulsed entry characterized by a transient overdose, followed by a relative short period of acceptable dosing, which is in turn followed by a prolonged period of under dosing. From a therapeutical point of view, inserts have been a success in the improvement of accurate dosing, and drug bioavailability and by the reduction of systemic absorption, and consequently side effects. However, the inserts are not well tolerated or accepted by patients, due to difficulties encountered in the application, psychological factors, and possible interference with vision.

Inserts were developed more than 30 years ago to treat the symptoms of dry eyes. Inserts dissolve and/or erode on contact with the ocular surface and therefore need to be used in addition with other artificial tears to initiate the dissolving process. Although the sustained release effect is very pronounced, insert use is severely diminished by the high cost, as well as the difficulty in handling inserts for elderly people, and the intense foreign body sensation.

Considering the various mucoadhesion mechanisms, hydration or degree of swelling of the polymers involved play an important role. In the case of dry or partially hydrated dosage forms, water movement from the mucus layer to the formulation can be a significant factor in mucoadhesion, being more important than molecular interpenetration. However, excessive water content leads to an abrupt drop in adhesive strength due to the formation of slippery non-adhesive mucilage at the interface. The contact time between the mucoadhesive dosage form and the mucus layer determines the extent of swelling and interpenetration of the polymer chains. The swelling time is important for the assessment of the adhesiveness. Decreasing the swelling time results in an improvement of the interpenetration phenomena. Hydrophilic polymers with poor mucoadhesive properties may be added to a mucoadhesive polymer with poor swelling characteristics to ensure fast swelling. Some additional polymers can hinder the formation of bonds between the mucoadhesive polymer and mucus by preferentially binding to the hydrated mucoadhesive polymer. There is also a reduction in the strength of the bond between the mucoadhesive polymer and mucin. During the last decade, notwithstanding the drawbacks encountered, and the low commercial success rate of inserts, but convinced about the therapeutical advantages offered by solid ocular dosage forms, many research groups directed their efforts to the development of better physiologically adapted and properly engineered devices with precise controlled drug release and bio/mucoadhesive properties[111-116].

Polymers used in Nanoscale Release Systems

Poly(esters)

The most studied and best characterized class of polymers for controlled release is the poly(esters). One of the most common polymers used in nanoparticle drug delivery approaches is poly(lactic-co-glycolic acid) (PLGA) due to its degradation properties, biocompatibility, and the fact that it is very well characterized[117]. PLGA degrades in an aqueous environment through the hydrolysis of the backbone ester linkages[118-119]. The polymeric device based on PLGA degrades through bulk erosion at a uniform rate throughout the matrix. The degradation process is self-catalyzed as the number of terminal carboxylic acid groups rises with increasing chain scission, and the acids catalyze the hydrolysis. The degradation is highly dependent on the ratio of lactide to glycolide moieties as lactide is more hydrophobic and reduces the rate of degradation[120]. Also, important factors in the degradation process are the degree of crystallinity, the molecular weight, and the glass transition temperature of the polymer. PLGA has been used to encapsulate a myriad of drugs and genes for controlled delivery applications for many diseases or other applications, and only a few are mentioned here. One popular area for the application of PLGA nanoparticles is in the treatment of cancer. Paclitaxel loaded nanoparticles (< 200 nm) with near 100% efficiency using an interfacial deposition method released approximately half of their payload within the first 24 hours and had a slowing release rate over the subsequent 4 days. Significant losses in viability were shown in the human small lung cancer cell line NCI-H69 with exposure to as little as 0.025 mg/ml paclitaxel-loaded nanoparticles[121]. Doxorubicin is a widely used cancer drug that impedes nucleic acid synthesis, yet is also known to have various systemic side effects. Nanoparticles prepared from PLGA–doxorubicin conjugates of about 200 nm in diameter suppressed tumor growth for 12 days after a single administration[122]. This is indicative of the ability of PLGA nanoparticles to control the release of drugs and be useful in sustaining release in a stent-like treatment without inducing systemic toxicity of these powerful drugs. Additional work has been accomplished in this area showing the promise of active targeting and the further utility of nanoparticles to prevent restenosis[123-124]. These studies show the utility of nanoparticles to sustain and spatially concentrate the delivery of an active agent in treatment of restenosis[125].

Poly (ortho esters)

Devices degrading through bulk erosion have an undesirable release profile for many applications, and the need for a device controlling release solely through hydrolysis of chains at the surface of the device effected the design of poly(ortho esters. The release rates from devices composed of poly(ortho esters) can be controlled by including acidic or basic excipients into the matrix as its hydrolysis is acid catalyzed. This has been used in the release of 5-fluorouracil[126], tetracycline[127], and others. Additionally, the mechanical properties of these polymers can be tailored by choosing from the various diols available.

Poly(anhydrides)

Poly(anhydrides) degrade by hydrolysis yet the polymer itself is hydrophobic in nature. These properties lead to surface erosion of the polymeric device and nearly zero-order release. The hydrolytic bond cleavage of poly(anhydrides) produces water-soluble products that in many cases are considered biocompatible. Poly(anhydrides) are most commonly produced through a melt-condensation polymerization. The most common polymers in this class are based on sebacic acid, p-(carboxyphenoxy) propane, and p–(carboxyphenoxy) hexane. Variations in monomer composition, such as hydrophobicity, influence the degradation rate of the polymeric device. The degradation can last from days to years depending on the composition. The photosensitizer phthalocyanine was chemically incorporated into nanoparticles based on biodegradable poly(sebacic anhydride)[128] for cancer treatment through photodynamic therapy. The attachment of the phthalocyanines to the polymer in the nanoparticles impedes the tendency of the agent to aggregate and become less useful for photodynamic therapy. The average hydrodynamic radius of the nanoparticles was found to be 166 nm. The release of photosensitizer from the particles was degradation dependent, and the rate of degradation increased with pH and temperature. This colloidal system has the potential to be useful for the delivery and controlled release of photosensitizer for photodynamic therapy. Many other types of poly(anhydrides) have been used in drug delivery applications in the nanoscale size range.

Cellulose Derivatives

The first cellulose polymer, methycellulose, was introduced over 50 years ago. Subsequently, a number of substituted cellulose-ethers have been employed for artificial tear solutions[129-130] and as viscosity-enhancing ophthalmic vehicles **(Figure 6.10)**. Methylcellulose also possesses wound healing properties and is a suitable tear substitute for dry eyes, especially for those with punctuate lesions[131]. All cellulose-ethers impart viscosity to the solution, have wetting properties and increase the contact time by virtue of film forming properties. Some cellulose-ethers (e.g. hydroxy-propylmethylcellulose and hydroxypropylcellulose) also exhibit surface active properties, interact with components of the tear film and alter the physicochemical parameters governing the tear film stability. Surface active viscosifying agents can influence the blinkingrate, which in turn influences the elimination of the drug instilled. They cause irritation and extensive lachrymation, provoking a rapid wash out of the ophthalmic solution and consequently a poor bioavailability. Generally, less surface active hydroxyethylcellulose is better tolerated, but the mucoadhesive properties of non-ionic cellulose-ethers are rather poor[132-133]. Sodium carboxymethylcellulose (NaCMC), however, exhibits a mucoadhesive capacity comparable to that of poly(acrylic acid) (PAA). Cationic cellulose derivatives (UcareR polymer JR 400), eventually in conjunction with anionic polymers (NaCMC, PAA, sodium hyaluronate), were proposed as sustained delivery systems of cationic therapeutic agents for the treatment of, for example, glaucoma[134]. From rheological data, it was deduced that the interactions between mucin and the JR 300 M derivative are mainly based on physical entanglement and less on ionic interactions[135].

Acrylates

The first mucoadhesive polymers proposed were poly(acrylic acid) and carbomers[136]. The mucoadhesive properties of poly(acrylic acid) are due mainly to hydrogen bonding, while hydrophobic interaction with mucin is not significant[137]. When anionic polymers interact with mucin, the maximum interactive adhesive force occurs at an acidic pH, suggesting that the mucoadhesive polymer in its protonated form is responsible for the mucoadhesion. The swollen polymer entangles with mucin on the eye surface, stabilizing a thick hydrogel structure[138]. In contrast, in the precorneal area, the neutral pH value of the tears and the shielding of the carboxyl groups by cations present in the tear fluid diminish the interaction of carbomer with the functional groups on mucin. A decrease in mucoadhesion is measured[139].

Rheological studies performed with various kinds of carbopolR (974P NF, 980 NF, 1342 NF) demonstrated no significant differences in the interaction between these different carbomers and mucin. It was demonstrated that the interaction depends on the mucin concentration, which implies that this interaction is only possible close to the corneal/conjunctival epithelium. Physical entanglement and secondary bond formation between poly(acrylic acid) derivatives and diluted mucin in the tear film can be excluded[140]. The use of non-neutralized polycarbophil, in order to prolong the precorneal residence time due to in situ gel formation and mucoadhesion, was proposed by Robinson and by Lehr et al.[141], whereas several researchers investigated poly(acrylic acid)– drug salts complexes in order to improve ocular bioavailability[142]. Polyanionic polymers such as polyacrylates or carbomers were proposed as long-lasting artificial tears for the relief of dry eye syndrome and traumatic injury. The use of these high molecular weight polymers is based on inherent mucuslike and lubricating properties, shear thinning behaviour, and good retention on the ocular surface[143]. Concentration-dependent blurring of vision and uncomfortable feeling are sometimes reported[144]. To enable the controlled release of drugs with low solubility, Setiawan et al. synthesized poly(acrylic acid)–cyclodextrin conjugates (Carbopol 934P:hydroxypropyl-beta-cyclodextrin). When administrated to the eye, an increase in the bioavailability of the drug complexed with cyclodextrin can be obtained. Moreover, after instillation, the preparation forms a gel. In rabbits, the aqueous humour bioavailability (as determined by the area under the concentration time profile over the first 3 h) of hydrocortisone 0.3% (w/v) in the new delivery system was 6-fold higher than for the suspension. A similar increase was observed for the cornea and the iris/ciliary body bioavailability[145].

Hyaluronan

Besides synthetic polymers, natural macromolecules such as hyaluronan (HA), present in the vitreous body of the eye, were proposed as viscosifying agents. Sodium hyaluronate molecules have physical properties and a composition comparable to tear glycoproteins, and easily coat the corneal epithelium. Polymers adsorbed at the mucin/aqueous interface extend into the adjacent aqueous phase, thereby stabilizing a thick layer of water. The non-Newtonian behaviour of sodium hyaluronate combines the advantage of high viscosity at rest between blinks with those of lower viscosity during blinking[146-147]. According to Chrai and Robinson, a pseudoplastic behaviour of an ophthalmic vehicle would be a disadvantage compared to a Newtonian solution which retains its viscosity during blinking. In the case of hyaluronans, the shear thinning characteristics do not seem to be disadvantageous, probably because of bioadhesive properties[148]. Diluted solutions of sodium hyaluronate have been employed successfully as tear substitutes in severe dry eye disorders. The beneficial effects are attributed to the viscoelasticity, biophysical properties similar to mucins, providing a long-lasting hydration and retention. Moreover, good lubrication of the ocular surface is obtained[149]. Hyaluronic acid is an important constituent of the extracellular matrix and may play a role in inflammation and wound healing and may promote corneal epithelial cell proliferation[150]. Gurny et al. confirmed the positive influence of hyaluronate vehicles on the bioavailability of pilocarpine[151]. High molecular weight of the polymer is an essential requirement for the prolonged precorneal residence time of the preparation[152-153].

Herrero-Vanrell *et al.* studied the effect of bioadhesive polymers on the bioavailability of tropicamide in rabbits. Drug solutions with NaCMC and poly (acrylic acid) resulted in mucoadhesion and mydriatic response, expressed as AUC0Y6 h, 1.9 and 1.4 times higher than the aqueous solution. Although the solution with sodium hyaluronate was less mucoadhesive than poly(acrylic acid), the hyaluronan preparation resulted in a higher AUC mydriasis/time value. The mydriatic effect remained up to 5.5 h for sodium hyaluronate and NaCMC[154]. Drug molecules not bound to the viscosifying agent can be squeezed out of the polymer network into the precorneal tear film during blinking. Camber and Lundgren demonstrated that small molecules diffuse without hindrance through the network[155]. Accordingly, some researchers proposed to bind the drug molecule to the polymer in order to slow down the drainage and to sustain the resorption. Bucolo and Mangiafico tested a formulation based on a pilocarpine hyaluronate salt in rabbits. An improved bioavailability, a 2-fold increase in miotic response and an extended duration of action were measured. Increased efficacy and duration of the therapeutic effect compared to a commercial preparation were obtained[156]. Another example of complex formation to improve ocular bioavailability consists of a ternary system of cationic drug (tetrazoline HCl), anionic polymer (hyaluronan) and gelatin[157].

Polysaccharides

Besides chitosan, numerous polysaccharides were evaluated as mucoadhesive ophthalmic vehicles: polygalacturonic acid, xyloglucan, xanthan gum, gellan gum, pullulan, guar gum, scleroglucan and carrageenan[158-161]. Also, in the case of polysaccharides, the formation of macromolecular ionic complexes with drugs improved the bioa - vailability and lengthened the therapeutic effect when compared to drug solutions[162].

Toxicological studies indicate that xyloglucan is very well tolerated by conjunctival cells, has cell protective properties and is able to reduce drug-related toxicity (e.g. fluoroquinolones, timolol, merthiolate) probably due to its mucin-like structure. Xyloglucan might promote wound healing depending on its influence on the integrin recognition system[163].

Timolol, in association with xyloglucan, has a prolonged duration of action, and is suitable for ocular administration in cases of elevated intraocular pressure[164]. In rabbits, high timolol concentrations in the ocular tissues were measured, but with low systemic absorption. The performances were comparable to the in situ gelling system of TimopticR XE containing gellan gum.

Xanthan Gum

Xanthan gum interacts moderately with mucin: a small viscoelastic synergistic effect can be observed, but the effect is due to physical entanglement of both components. Xanthan gum should exist as an ordered double-stranded helix in the precorneal tear film, due to ions present in the lacrimal fluid[165]. Results of an *in vivo* study in healthy volunteers confirm that an increase in viscosity of xanthan gum solutions delays the clearance of the instilled solution. Xanthan gum is therefore more suitable as a viscosifying agent when compared to poly(vinyl alcohol), hydroxyethylcellulose and hydroxypropylmethyl cellulose. However, the effect of the gelation mechanism of gellan gum is superior compared to xanthan gum, especially at the later time points[166].

Cellulose
R: H (cellulose) CH_3 (methylcellulose) CH_2COONa (sodium carboxymethylcellulose) CH_3 and OCH_2CH (OH) CH_3 (hydroxypropylemethylcellulose) $CH_2CH_2OCH_2CH_2OH$ (hydroxyethylcellulose)
Hyaluronic acid	
Chitosan	
Alginic acid	
Xanthan gum	

Gellan gum	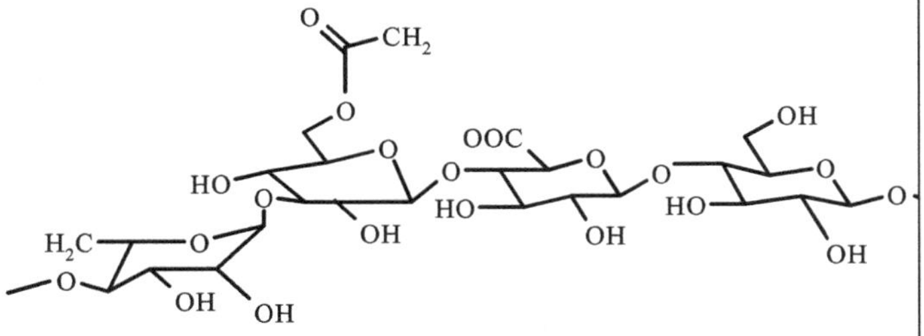
PAA	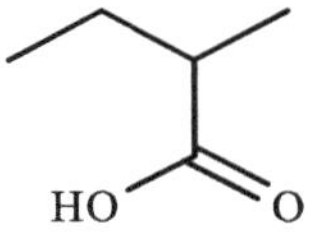
Eudragit RS, RL	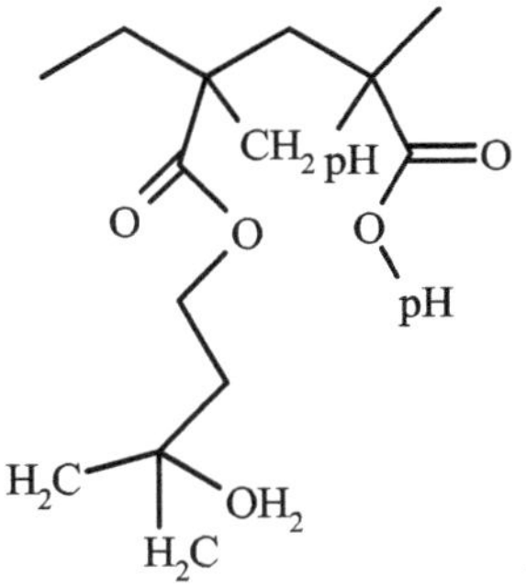 R1 : H CH₃ R2 : CH3, C₂H₅
PACA	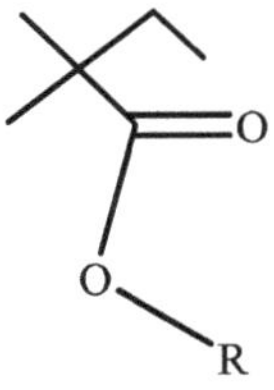 R : Methyl (PMCA) Ethyl (PECA) Butyl (PBCA) Isobutyl (PIBCA) Hyxyl (PHCA)

Fig. 6.10 Chemical structure of cellulose derivatives and polymers.

Thiomers

In order to significantly improve mucoadhesion, poly(acrylates), chitosan, alginate, deacetylated gellan gum and cellulose derivatives were synthesized with immobilized thiol groups (e.g. l-cysteine) **(Figure 6.11)** by Bernkop-Schnuerch et al.[167]. The rationale of the concept is based on knowledge concerning the role of disulfide bridges in the three-dimensional mucin network formation. Thiolated polymers, or socalled thiomers, are capable of forming covalent bonds with cysteine-rich subdomains of mucins, whereas mucoadhesive polymers discussed so far formed non-covalent bonds (hydrogen bonds or ionic interactions) with mucus, or exhibited physical entanglements[168]. The extensive cross-linkingprocess of the thiomers with mucins resulted in a tremendous increase in viscosity and mucoadhesion independent of pH or ionic strength of the medium. The mucoadhesive properties of a chitosan thioglycolicm acid conjugate and a poly(acrylic acid)–cysteine conjugate improved 10-fold and even 100-fold, respectively, compare to the native polymers[169]. Cohesive properties of thiomers are improved as a simple oxidation process in aqueous media leads to the formation of inter- and/or intrachain disulfide bonds within the network. It has also been demonstrated that thiomers possess permeation enhancing properties for the paracellular uptake of drugs[170]. The mechanism is based on the opening of the tight junctions. The cysteine moieties of the thiomers are able to reduce oxidized glutathione and, therefore, the concentration of reduced glutathione on the absorption membrane is increased. Glutathione inhibits the enzyme protein–tyrosine–phosphatase, which leads to the phosphorylation of the membrane protein occludin, resulting in the opening of the tight junctions[171]. An in vitro study on the cornea of rabbits with polycarbophil–cysteine showed a 2.2-fold and 2.4- fold increase in the transcorneal permeation of sodium fluorescein and dexamethasone phosphate, respectively, when compared to the unmodified polycarbophil. No toxic effect was observed on the cornea of rabbits[172]. As a consequence of the in situ gelling and mucoadhesive properties of thiomers, a prolonged residence of the formulation and subsequently a prolonged time period of drug absorption are achieved. The permeation enhancing properties will further improve bioavailability of incorporated drugs. When water-soluble polymers are cross-linked, the mobility of individual polymer chains decreases. The effective length of the chain that penetrates into the mucus layer also decreases, which can reduce mucoadhesive strength. Cross-linking or covalent attachment of large sized ligands leads to reduction in chain flexibility and results in a strong decrease in mucoadhesion. Leitner et al. demonstrated that low molecular mass polymers with flexible chains favouring strong interpenetration are not cohesive enough for optimal mucoadhesion, whereas high molecular weight cross-linked polymers showing high cohesiveness do not display enough chain flexibility[173]. Thus, the right choice of the polymer during the development of ophthalmic delivery systems, taking into account the site of administration, will be essential. Free radical formation and inflammation are involved in dry eye pathology[174]. Thiomers could be useful additives in artificial tear formulation due to antioxidative and radical scavenging properties. Moreover, thiomers are similar to ocular mucins displaying numerous thiol groups. Thiomers could mimic the physiological process of the mucus layer such as tear film stabilization. The formation of disulfide bonds with mucins leads to strong mucoadhesion, prolonged residence time and protective effect for the corneal/conjunctival epithelium.

Chitosan cysteine	
Chitosan thioglycolic acid	

NaCMC cysteine	
Polyacrylic acid cysteine	

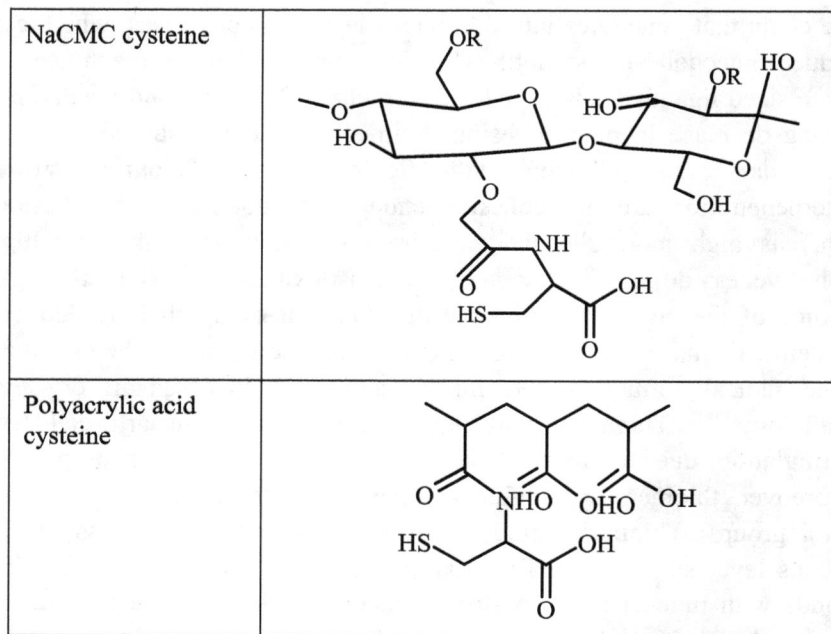

Fig. 6.11 Chemical structure of thiomers.

Chitosan

Chitosan is a naturally derived polysaccharide created by the deacetylation of chitin. The advantageous properties of chitosan include its biocompatibility, positive charge, the abundance of amine groups available for crosslinking, ease of processing, mucoadhesiveness, and its degradation into amino sugars, which are all attractive for drug delivery applications[175]. Chitosan nanoparticles have been formulated by a variety of techniques including emulsion crosslinking, complex coacervation, emulsion droplet coalescence method, ionic gelation, ionotropic gelation, and the reverse micellar method. The molecular weight of the chitosan, its degree of deacetylation, the extent of crosslinking, and its interactions with the encapsulated molecule play a role in controlling the release of the therapeutic agent from the particle. Due to its charge, the pH of the release media also influences release from chitosan particles. Release from chitosan particles occurs through similar mechanisms as mentioned for other particles: desorption of surface-adhered drug, diffusion through a swollen rubbery polymer matrix, and release due to erosion. Release of drugs from surface layers of the matrix involves a large burst effect, but increasing the crosslinking density can reduce this effect. Diffusion out of the matrix occurs through a three-step process: diffusion of water into the matrix causing swelling, transition from glassy to rubbery polymer, and diffusion of drug out of the matrix. The release follows a typical hydrogel release profile. Chitosan nanoparticles of approximately 100 nm in diameter prepared by a microemulsion method have been used to encapsulate a doxorubicin–dextran conjugate. In a mouse model, tumor volume was reduced after four weekly injections of the nanoparticle formulation 40% more than in mice treated with the conjugate alone, and injection of drug alone had no effect over control conditions[176]. As an adjuvant to another cancer therapy–neutron-capture therapy–gadopentetic acid (Gd-DTPA) has been loaded in chitosan nanoparticles formed by an emulsion droplet coalescence technique. Less than 2% of the Gd-DTPA was released over 7 days in PBS, but over 90% was released in plasma over 1 day. After an intratumoral injection in a mouse melanoma model, 92% of the Gd-DTPA was contained within the tumor site compared to only 1.2% of the Gd-DTPA injected in a non-nanoparticle formulation[177]. The Gd-DTPA chitosan nanoparticles have been shown to have a high affinity for uptake in several cell types, suggesting the mechanism for high retention in tumor[178].

Gelatin

Gelatin is a naturally occurring biopolymer that is biocompatible and biodegradable. The polymer is obtained through heat-dissolution and partial hydrolysis of collagen obtained from animal connective tissues. It has been used for many years in pharmaceutical applications such as capsules and ointments as well as early nanoformulations[179]. Recently, gelatin nanoparticles made by a two-step desolvation process involving crosslinking of the polymer using gluteraldehyde have been used to entrap cycloheximide, a protein synthesis inhibitor used in cancer treatment. Cycloheximide was entrapped with 26% efficiency in nanoparticles of 168 nm diameter. The particles were stable in whole blood, and they showed anti-tumor activity in two breast cancer cell lines over a period of time. The release kinetics curve was interestingly biphasic, and release was relatively slow. The gelatin nanoparticles are reportedly a good candidate for biopharmaceutical delivery[180]. Zwiorek et al. produced gelatin nanoparticles by the same desolvation method as a carrier for plasmid DNA. The particles were cationized in order to have an electrostatic interaction with the DNA which bounds onto the surface of the particles. The nanoparticles showed little cytotoxic effect, and efficient gene transfection was exhibited by an exponential increase in gene expression in B16 F10 cells.

Mechanisms of Mucoadhesion
(The Mucoadhesive / Mucosa Interaction)

Chemical Bonds

For adhesion to occur, molecules must bond across the interface. These bonds can arise in the following way[181].

1. **Ionic bonds**—where two oppositely charged ions attract each other via electrostatic interactions to form a strong bond (e.g. in a salt crystal).

2. **Covalent bonds**—where electrons are shared, in pairs, between the bonded atoms in order to dfillT the orbitals in both. These are also strong bonds.

3. **Hydrogen bonds**—here a hydrogen atom, when covalently bonded to electronegative atoms such as oxygen, fluorine or nitrogen, carries a slight positively charge and is therefore is attracted to other electronegative atoms. The hydrogen can therefore be thought of as being shared, and the bond formed is generally weaker than ionic or covalent bonds.

4. **Van-der-Waals bonds**—these are some of the weakest forms of interaction that arise from dipole–dipole and dipole-induced dipole attractions in polar molecules, and dispersion forces with non-polar substances.

5. **Hydrophobic bonds**—more accurately described as the hydrophobic effect, these are indirect bonds (such groups only appear to be attracted to each other) that occur when non-polar groups are present in an aqueous solution. Water molecules adjacent to non-polar groups form hydrogen bonded structures, which lowers the system entropy. There is therefore an increase in the tendency of non-polar groups to associate with each other to minimise this effect.

Theories of Adhesion

There are six general theories of adhesion, which have been adapted for the investigation of mucoadhesion[182-183]. The electronic theory suggests that electron transfer occurs upon contact of adhering surfaces due to differences in their electronic structure. This is proposed to result in the formation of an electrical double layer at the interface, with subsequent adhesion due to attractive forces. The wetting theory is primarily applied to liquid systems and considers surface and interfacial energies. It involves the ability of a liquid to spread spontaneously onto a surface as a prerequisite for the development of adhesion. The affinity of a liquid for a surface can be found using techniques such as contact angle goniometry to measure the contact angle of the liquid on the surface, with the general rule being that the lower the contact angle, the greater the affinity of the liquid to the solid. The spreading coefficient (S_{AB}) can be calculated from the surface energies of the solid and liquids using the equation:

$$S_{AB} = \gamma_B - \gamma_A - \gamma_{AB}$$

where γ_A is the surface tension (energy) of the liquid A, γ_B is the surface energy of the solid B and cAB is the interfacial energy between the solid and liquid. S_{AB} should be positive for the liquid to spread spontaneously over the solid.

The work of adhesion (WA) represents the energy required to separate the two phases, and is given by:

$$WA = \gamma_{A +} \gamma_{A -} \gamma_{AB}$$

The greater the individual surface energies of the solid and liquid relative to the interfacial energy, the greater the work of adhesion. The adsorption theory describes the attachment of adhesives on the basis of hydrogen bonding and van der Waals' forces. It has been proposed that these forces are the main contributors to the adhesive interaction. A subsection of this, the chemisorptions theory, assumes an interaction across the interface occurs as a result of strong covalent bonding.

The diffusion theory describes interdiffusion of polymers chains across an adhesive interface. This process is driven by concentration gradients and is affected by the available molecular chain lengths and their mobilities. The depth of interpenetration depends on the diffusion coefficient and the time of contact. Sufficient depth of penetration creates a semi-permanent adhesive bond.

The mechanical theory assumes that adhesion arises from an interlocking of a liquid adhesive (onsetting) into irregularities on a rough surface. However, rough surfaces also provide an increased surface area available for interaction along with an enhanced viscoelastic and plastic dissipation of energy during joint failure, which are thought to be more important in the adhesion process than a mechanical effect. The fracture theory differs a little from the other five in that it relates the adhesive strength to the forces required for the detachment of the two involved surfaces after adhesion. This assumes that the failure of the adhesive bond occurs at the interface. However, failure normally occurs at the weakest component, which is typically a cohesive failure within one of the adhering surfaces.

Various Theories of Mucoadhesion

Due its relative complexity, it is likely that the process of mucoadhesion cannot be described by just one of these theories. In considering the mechanism of mucoadhesion, a whole range 'scenarios' for in-vivo mucoadhesive bond formation are possible (**Figure 6.12**).

These include:

1. Dry or partially hydrated dosage forms contacting surfaces with substantial mucus layers (typically particulates administered into the nasal cavity).

2. Fully hydrated dosage forms contacting surfaces with substantial mucus layers (typically particulates of many 'First Generation' mucoadhesives that have hydrated in the luminal contents on delivery to the lower gastrointestinal tract).

3. Dry or partially hydrated dosage forms contacting surfaces with thin/discontinuous mucus layers (typically tablets or patches in the oral cavity or vagina).

4. Fully hydrated dosage forms contacting surfaces with thin/discontinuous mucus layers (typically aqueous semisolids or liquids administered into the oesophagus or eye).

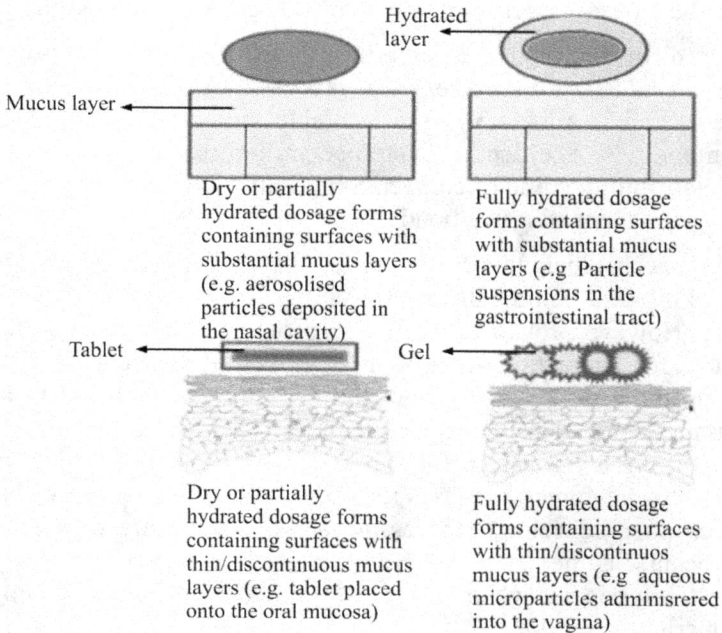

Fig. 6.12 Some scenarios of mucoadhesion.

It is unlikely that the mucoadhesive process will be the same in each case. In the study of adhesion generally, two steps in the adhesive process have been identified[184], which have been adapted to describe the interaction between mucoadhesive materials and a mucous membrane **(Figure 6.13).**

Step 1 —Contact stage: An intimate contact (wetting) occurs between the mucoadhesive and mucous membrane.

Step 2 —Consolidation stage: Various physicochemical interactions occur to consolidate and strengthen the adhesive joint, leading to prolonged adhesion.

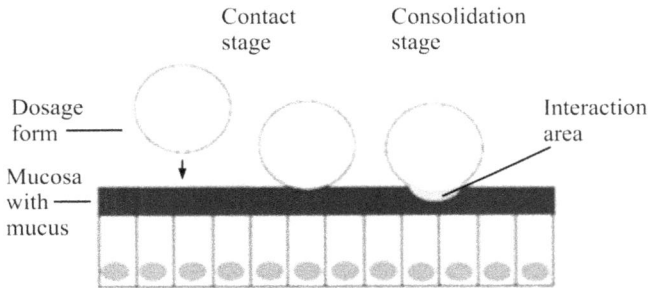

Fig. 6.13 The two stages in mucoadhesion.

However, when a substantial mucus layer is present then the anti-adherent properties of mucus will need to be overcome if a strong adhesive joint is to be formed. In this case the adhesive joint can be considered to contain three regions **(Figure 6.14)**, the mucoadhesive, the mucosa and an interfacial region, consisting at least initially of mucus. To achieve strong adhesion, a change in the physical properties of the mucus layer will be required otherwise it will readily fail on application of a dislodging stress.

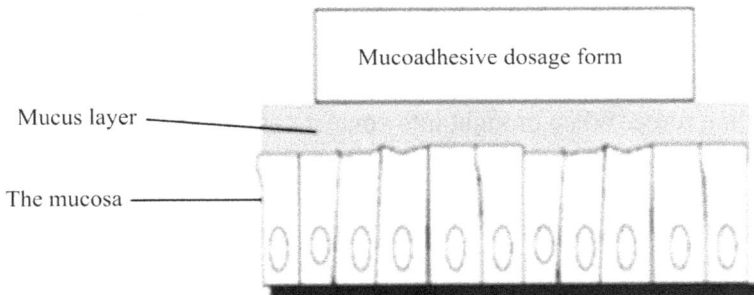

Fig. 6.14 The three regiosns within a mucoadhesive joint.

There are essentially two theories as to how gel strengthening/ consolidation occurs. One is based on a macromolecular interpenetration effect, which has been dealt with in a theoretical basis by Peppas and Sahlin. In this theory, based largely on the diffusion theory described by Voyutskii for compatible polymeric systems, the mucoadhesive molecules interpenetrate and bond by secondary interactions with mucus glycoproteins **(Figure 6.15).** Evidence for this is provided by an ATIR FTIR study by Jabbari et al.

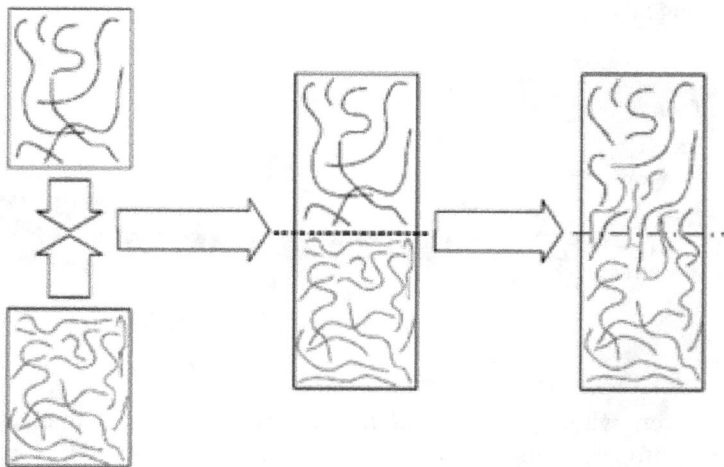

Fig. 6.15 The interpenetration theory; three stages in the interaction between a mucoadhesive polymer and mucin glycoprotein.

The second theory is the dehydration theory. When a material capable of rapid gelation in an aqueous environment is brought into contact with a second gel water movement occurs between gels until equilibrium is achieved. A polyelectrolyte gel, such as a poly(acrylic acid) will have a strong affinity for water, therefore a high dosmotic pressureT and a large swelling force. When brought into contact with a mucus gel it will rapidly dehydrate that gel and force intermixing and consolidation of the mucus joint **(Figure 6.16)** until equilibrium is reached. The movement of water from mucus into a poly(acrylic acid) film was observed by Jabbari et al. A mucus gel, on dehydration, goes from having lubricant to the opposite adhesive properties, as observed in studies by Mortazavi and Smart.

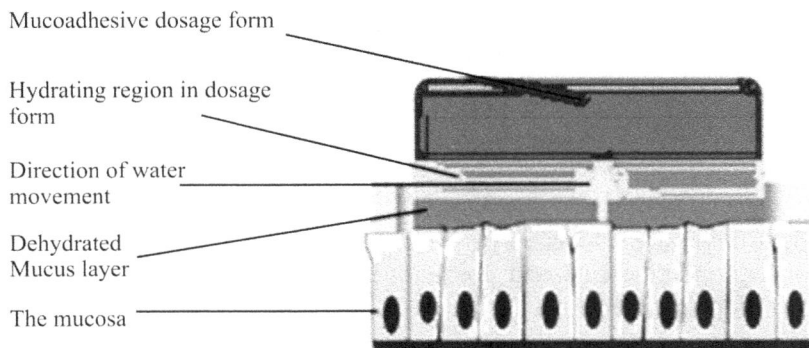

Mucoadhesive dosage form

Hydrating region in dosage form

Direction of water movement

Dehydrated Mucus layer

The mucosa

Fig. 6.16 The dehydration theory of mucoadhesion.

Removal mechanisms: Adhesive failure will normally occur at the weakest component of the joint **(Figure 6.17)**. For weaker adhesives this would be the mucoadhesive–mucus interface, for stronger adhesives this would initially be the mucus layer, but later may be the hydrating mucoadhesive material[185]. On application of a constant tensile stress to compacts of mucoadhesive polymers, joint failure was found by Mortazavi and Smart[186] to be a cohesive failure of the swelling polymer for all but the weakest adhesives. The strength and durability of the adhesive joint will therefore depend on the cohesive nature of the weakest region. The mucoadhesive polymer in an aqueous environment can overhydrate to form slippery mucilage, which is readily removed. Controlling the rate and extent of hydration is required to produce prolonged adhesion and strategies such as cross-linking[187-188] and introducing hydrophobic entities[189] has been tried to achieve this. In all cases, eventually all formulations will be displaced by mucus or cell turnover[190-192].

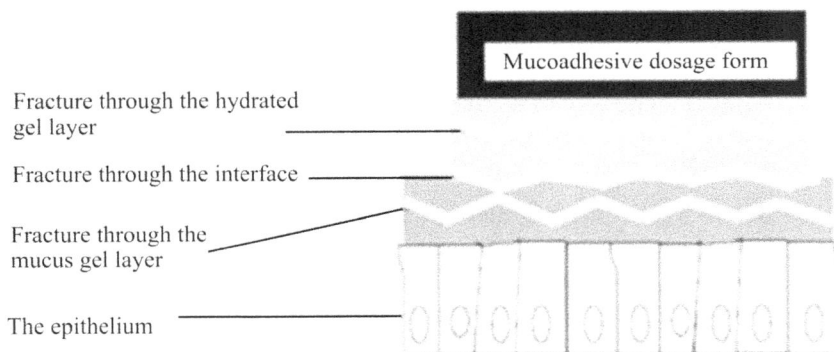

Mucoadhesive dosage form

Fracture through the hydrated gel layer

Fracture through the interface

Fracture through the mucus gel layer

The epithelium

Fig. 6.17 The possible regions for mucoadhesive failure.

References

1. Mehnert W and K Mader, Solid lipid nanoparticles: Production, characterization and applications, Adv Drug Deliv Rev, 2001, 47, 165-196.

2. Walde P, Ichikawa S, Enzymes inside lipid vesicles: preparation, reactivity and applications, Biomol Eng, 2001, 18, 143–77.

3. Couvreur P, Dubernet C, Puisieux F, Controlled drug delivery with nanoparticles: current possibilities and future trends, Eur J Pharm Biopharm, 1995, 41, 2–13.

4. Couvreur P, Kante B, Roland M, Polycyanoacrylate nanocapsules as potential lysosomotropic carriers: preparation, morphological and sorptive properties, J Pharm Pharmacol, 1979, 31, 331–332.

5. Durrani A M, Davies N M, Thomas M, Kellaway I W, Pilocarpine bioavailability from a mucoadhesive liposomal ophthalmic drug delivery system, Int J Pharm, 1992, 88, 409-415.

6. Fendler JH, Fendler EJ, Catalysis in Micellar and Macromolecular Systems, Academic Press, New York, 1975.

7. Agostiano A, Catalano M, Curri ML, Della Monica M, Manna L, Vasanelli L, Synthesis and structural characterisation of CdS nanoparticles prepared in a four-components "water-in-oil" microemulsion, Micron, 2000, 31, 253-258.

8. Fang J, Stokes KL, Wiemann JA, Zhou WL, Dia ZJ, Microemulsion processed bismuth nanoparticles, Mat Sci Eng, 2001, B83, 254-257.

9. Zara GP, bargoni A, Cavalli R, Fundaro A, Vighetto D, Gasco MR, Pharmacokinetic and tissue distribution of idarubicin- loaded solid lipid nanoparticles after duodenal administration to rats, J pharm Sci, 2002, 91, 1324-1333.

10. Kipp JE, The role of solid nanoparticle technology in the parenteral delivery of poorly water-soluble drugs, Int J Pharm, 2004, 284, 109–122.

11. Setler P, Identifying new oral technologies to meet your drug delivery needs for the delivery of peptides and proteins and poorly soluble molecules. IIR Limited Drug Delivery Systems, London, March 1999.

12. Liversidge GG and Cundy KC, Particle size reduction for improvement of oral bioavailability of hydrophobic drugs, Int J Pharm, 1995, 125, 91–97.

13. Knight P, Transforming potential for difficult drugs, Drug Delivery, 2006, 6–8.

14. Hu J, Johnston KP, Williams RO, Nanoparticle engineering process for enhancing the dissolution rates of poorly water soluble drugs, Drug Dev Ind Pharm, 2004, 30, 233–245.

15. Muller RH, Jacobs C, Kayser O, Nanosuspension as particulate drug formulations in therapy rationale for development and what we can expect for the future, Adv Drug Deliv Rev, 2001, 47, 3–19.

16. Dearn AR, Atovaquone pharmaceutical compositions. European patent EU 0/075711, 1995

17. Lockman PR, Mumper RJ, Khan MA, Allen DD, Nanoparticle technology for drug delivery across the blood-brain barrier, Drug Dev Ind Pharm, 2002, 28.

18. Feng S, Nanoparticles of biodegradable polymers for new-concept chemotherapy, Expert Rev Med Devices, 2004, 1, 115–125

19. Oyewumi MO and Mumper RJ, Gadolinium loaded nanoparticles engineered from microemulsion templates, Drug Dev Ind Pharm, 2002, 28, 317–328.

20. Mehnert W and Mader K, Solid lipid nanoparticles: production, characterization and applications, Adv Drug Del Rev, 2001, 47, 165–196.

21. Gasco MR, Solid lipid nanospheres from warm microemulsions, Pharm Tech Eur, 1997, 9, 52–58.

22. Mumper RJ, Cui Z, Oyewumi MO, Nanotemplate engineering of cellspecific nanoparticles, J Disp Sci Tech, 2003, 24, 569–588.

23. Ferrari M, Cancer nanotechnology: Opportunities and challenges, Nat. Rev. Cancer, 2005, 5, 161.

24. Brigger I, Dubernet C, Couvreur P, Nanoparticles in cancer therapy and diagnosis, Adv Drug Deliv Rev, 2002, 54, 631.

25. Kobayashi H. and Brechbiel MW, Dendrimer-based macromolecular MRI contrast agents: Characteristics and application, Mol Imaging, 2003, 2, 1–10.

26. Cole C, Tumor-targeted, systemic delivery of therapeutic viral vectors using hitchhiking on antigen-specific T cells, Nat Med, 2005, 11, 1073–1081.

27. Voura EB, Tracking metastatic tumor cell extravasation with quantum dot nanocrystals and fluorescence emission-scanning microscopy, Nat Med, 2004, 10, 993–998.

28. Bianco A, Kostarelos K, Biomedical applications of functionalised carbon nanotubes, Chemical Communications, 2005b, 5, 571–577.

29. Ajima K and Yudasaka M, Carbon nanohorns as anticancer drug carriers, Molecular Pharmacology, 2005, 2, 475–480.

30. Iijima S, Helical microtubules of graphitic carbon, Nature, 1991, 354, 56–58.

31. Iijima S. and Ichihashi T, Single-shell carbon nanotubes of 1-nm diameter, Nature, 1993, 363, 603–605.

32. Lam CW, James JT, Pulmonary Toxicity of Single-Wall Carbon Nanotubes in Mice 7 and 90 Days After Intratracheal Instillation, 2004, 77, 126–134.

33. Whitesides GM, Mathias JP, Molecular self-assembly and nanochemistry: a chemical strategy for the synthesis of nanostructures, Science, 1991, 254: 1312–1319.

34. Zhu HW, Xu CL, Direct Synthesis of Long Single-Walled Carbon Nanotube Strands, 2002, 296, 884–886.

35. Dresselhaus MDG and Eklund PC, Science of Fullerenes and Carbon Nanotubes, San Diego, 1996a, Academic Press, Inc.

36. Klumpp C, Kostarelos K, Functionalized carbon nanotubes as emerging nanovectors for the delivery of therapeutics, Biochimica et Biophysica Acta-Biomembranes, 2006, 1758, 404–412.

37. Balasubramanian, K. and M. Burghard, Chemically functionalized carbon nanotubes, Small, 2005, 1, 180–192.

38. Dresselhaus MDG, Eklund PC, Science of Fullerenes and Carbon Nanotubes, San Diego, 1996a, Academic Press, Inc.

39. Lu JP, Elastic Properties of Carbon Nanotubes and Nanoropes, Physical Review Letters, 1997, 79, 1297.

40. Haddon RC, Carbon Nanotubes, Acc Chem Res, 2002, 35, 12.

41. Hone J, Batlogg B, Quantized Phonon Spectrum of Single-Wall Carbon Nanotubes, 2002, 289, 1730–1733.

42. Sun YP, Fu K, Functionalized Carbon Nanotubes: Properties and Applications, Accounts of Chemical Research, 2002, 35, 1096–1104.

43. Bianco A, Hoebeke J, Carbon nanotubes: on the road to deliver, Current Drug Delivery, 2005a, 2, 253–259.

44. Jain KK, The role of nanobiotechnology in drug discovery, Drug Discovery Today, 2005, 10, 1435–1442.

45. Shim M, Kam NWS, Functionalization of carbon nanotubes for biocompatibility and biomolecular recognition, Nano Letters, 2002, 2, 285–288.

46. Vasir JK, Reddy MK, Nanosystems in drug targeting: Opportunities and challenges, Current Nanoscience, 2005, 1, 47–64.

47. Shvedova A, Castranova V, Exposure to Carbon Nanotube Material: Assessment of Nanotube Cytotoxicity using Human Keratinocyte Cells, J Toxicol and Env Health Part A, 2003, 66, 1909–1926.

48. Salvador-Morales C, Flahaut E, Complement activation and protein adsorption by carbon nanotubes, Molecular Immunology, 2006, 43, 193–201.

49. Bauer LA and Birenbaum NS, Biological applications of high aspect ratio nanoparticles, J Mat Chem, 2004, 14, 517–526.

50. Whitney T and Jiang JS, Fabrication and Magnetic Properties of Arrays of Metallic Nanowires, Science, 1993, 261, 1316–1319.

51. Salem AK, Directed assembly of multisegment Au/Pt/Au nanowires, Nano Letters, 2004, 4, 1163–1165.

52. Glomm WR, Functionalized gold nanoparticles for applications in bionanotechnology, J Dis Sci and Tech, 2005, 26, 389–414.

53. Huang K, Preparation of highly conductive, self-assembled gold/ polyaniline nanocables and polyaniline nanotubes, Chemistry-a European Journal, 2006, 12, 5314–5319.

54. Sun YP, Fu K, Functionalized Carbon Nanotubes: Properties and Applications, Accounts of Chem Res, 2002, 35, 1096–1104.

55. Salem AK, Hung CF, Multi-component nanorods for vaccination applications, Nanotechnology, 2005, 16, 484–487.

56. Nishikawa M, Targeted delivery of plasmid DNA to hepatocytes in vivo: Optimization of the pharmacokinetics of plasmid DNA galactosylated poly(L-lysine) complexes by controlling their physicochemical properties, J Pharmacol and Exp Therap, 1998, 287, 408–415.

57. Gaur U and Sahoo SK, Biodistribution of fluoresceinated dextran using novel nanoparticles evading reticuloendothelial system, Int J Pharm, 2000, 202, 1–10.

58. Venugopal J. and Ramakrishna S, Applications of polymer nanofibers in biomedicine and biotechnology, Applied Biochem and Biotech, 2005, 125, 147–157.

59. Thandavamoorthy S and Gopinath N, Self-assembled honeycomb polyurethane nanofibers, J Applied Polymer Sci, 2006, 101, 3121–3124.

60. Moghimi SM and Hunter AC, Nanomedicine: current status and future prospects, Faseb Journal, 2005, 19, 311–330.

61. Service RF, Nanofibers seed blood vessels, Science, 2005, 308, 44–45.

62. Greiner A and Wendorff JH, Biohybrid nanosystems with polymer nanofibers and nanotubes, Applied Microbiol and Biotechn, 2006, 71, 387–393.

63. He CL, Huang ZM, Coaxial electrospun poly(L-lactic acid) ultrafine fibers for sustained drug delivery, J Macromol Sci Part B-Physics, 2006, 45, 515–524.

64. Ma ZW, Kotaki M, Potential of nanofiber matrix as tissueengineering scaffolds, Tissue Engineering, 2005, 11, 101–109.

65. Jin HJ, Chen JS, Karageorgiou V, Altman GH, Kaplan DL, Human bone marrow stromal cell responses on electrospun silk fibroin mats, Biomaterials, 2004, 25, 1039.

66. Dresselhaus MS, Dresselhaus G, Eklund PC, Science of Fullerenes and Carbon Nanotubes, San Diego, 1996b, CA, Academic Press, Inc.

67. Dresselhaus MS, Dresselhaus G, Eklund PC, Science of Fullerenes and Carbon Nanotubes, San Diego, 1996b, CA, Academic Press, Inc.

68. Vogelson CT, Advances in drug delivery systems, Modern Drug Discovery, 2001, 4, 49–52.

69. Tegos GP, Demidova TN, Cationic Fullerenes Are Effective and Selective Antimicrobial Photosensitizers, Chemistry & Biology, 2005, 12, 1127–1135.

70. Tropin TV, Avdeev MV, Nonmonotonic behavior of the concentration in the kinetics of dissolution of fullerenes, Jetp Letters, 2006, 83, 399–404.

71. Leary SP, Liu CY, Toward the emergence of nanoneurosurgeryPart III – Nanomedicine: Targeted nanotherapy, nanosurgery, and progress toward the realization of nanoneurosurgery, Neurosurgery, 2006, 58, 1009–1025.

72. Dugan LLTD, Du C, Lobner D, Wheeler M, Almli CR, Shen CK-F, Luh T-Y Choi DW, Lin T-S, Carboxyfullerenes as neuroprotective agents, Proceedings of the National Academy of Sciences USA, 1997, 94, 9434–9439.

73. Chu LY, Liang YJ, Chen WM, Ju XJ, Wang HD, Preparation of glucose-sensitive microcapsules with a porous membrane and functional gates, Colloids Surf. B: Biointerfaces, 2004, 37, 9–14.

74. Kim JJ, and Park K, Modulated insulin delivery from glucose-sensitive hydrogel dosage forms, J Control Release, 2001, 77, 39–47.

75. Lee ES, Shin HJ, Na K, Bae YH, Poly(L-histidine)-PEG block copolymer micelles and pH-induced destabilization, J Control Release, 2003, 90, 363–374.

76. Lee ES, Na K, Bae YH, Super pH-sensitive multifunctional polymeric micelle, Nano Lett, 2005b, 5, 325–329.

77. Hruby M, Konak C, Ulbrich K, Polymeric micellar pH-sensitive drug delivery system for doxorubicin, J Control Release, 2005, 103, 137–148.

78. Ringsdorf H, Structure and properties of pharmacologically active polymers, J Polym Sci Polym Sympo, 1975, 51, 135–153.

79. Duncan R, Polymer conjugates as anticancer nanomedicines, Nat Rev Cancer, 2006, 6, 688–701.

80. Ho YP, Chen HH, Leong KW, Wang TH, Evaluating the intracellular stability and unpacking of DNA nanocomplexes by quantum dots- FRET, J Control Release, 2006, 116, 83–89.

81. Davis FF, The origin of pegnology, Adv Drug Deliv Rev, 2002, 54, 457–468.

82. Chytil P, Etrych T, Konak C, Sirova M, Mrkvan T, Rihova B, Ulbrich K, Properties of HPMA copolymer-doxorubicin conjugates with pH-controlled activation: effect of polymer chain modification, J Control Release, 2006, 115, 26–36.

83. Gao SQ, Lu ZR, Petri B, Kopeckova P, Kopecek J, Colonspecific 9-aminocamptothecin-HPMA copolymer conjugates containing a 1,6- elimination spacer, J Control Release, 2006, 110, 323–331.

84. Greco F, Vicent MJ, Gee S, Jones AT, Gee J, Nicholson RI, Duncan R, Investigating the mechanism of enhanced cytotoxicity of HPMA copolymer-Dox-AGM in breast cancer cells, J Control Release, 2007, 11, 28–39.

85. Duncan R, Lloyd JB, Kopecek J, Degradation of side chains of N-(2- hydroxypropyl) methacrylamide copolymers by lysosomal enzymes, Biochem Biophys Res Commun, 1980, 94, 284–290.

86. Shimoboji T, Larenas E, Fowler T, Kulkarni S, Hoffman AS, Stayton PS, Photoresponsive polymer-enzyme switches, Proc Natl Acad Sci U S A, 2002, 99, 16592–16596.

87. Shimoboji T, Larenas E, Fowler T, Hoffman AS, Stayton PS, Temperature-induced switching of enzyme activity with smart polymer-enzyme conjugates, Bioconjug Chem, 2003, 14, 517–525.

88. Torchilin VP, Multifunctional nanocarriers, Adv Drug Deliv Rev, 2006, 58, 1532–1555.

89. Lukyanov AN, Elbayoumi TA, Chakilam AR, Torchilin VP, Tumor-targeted liposomes: doxorubicin-loaded long-circulating liposomes modified with anti-cancer antibody, J Control Release, 2004, 100, 135–144.

90. Sawant RM, Hurley JP, Salmaso S, Kale A, Tolcheva E, Levchenko TS, Torchilin VP, SMART drug delivery systems: double-targeted pHresponsive pharmaceutical nanocarriers, Bioconjug Chem, 2006, 17, 943–949.

91. Demello AJ, Control and detection of chemical reactions in microfluidic systems, Nature, 2006, 442, 394–402.

92. Janasek D, Franzke J, Manz A, Scaling and the design of miniaturized chemical-analysis systems, Nature, 2006, 442, 374–380.

93. Psaltis D, Quake SR, Yang C, Developing optofluidic technology through the fusion of microfluidics and optics, Nature, 2006, 442, 381–386.

94. Whitesides GM, The origins and the future of microfluidics, Nature, 2006, 442, 368–373.

95. Yager P, Edwards T, Fu E, Helton K, Nelson K, Tam MR, Weigl BH, Microfluidic diagnostic technologies for global public health, Nature, 2006, 442, 412–418.

96. Maloney JM, Uhland SA, Polito BF, Sheppard NF, Jr Pelta CM, Santini JT, Electrothermally activated microchips for implantable drug delivery and biosensing, J Control Release, 2005, 109, 244–255.

97. Tao SL, and Desai TA, Micromachined devices: the impact of controlled geometry from cell-targeting to bioavailability, J Control Release, 2005, 109, 127–138.

98. Richards Grayson AC, Scheidt Shawgo R, Li Y, Cima MJ, Electronic MEMS for triggered delivery, Adv Drug Deliv Rev, 2004, 56, 173–184.

99. Baldi A, Gu Y, Loftness P, Siegel RA, Ziaie B, A hydrogelactuated environmentally-sensitive microvalve for active flow control, J Microelectromechanical Syst, 2003, 12, 613–621.

100. Goldstein D, Nassar T, Lambert G, Kadouche J, Benita S, The design and evaluation of a novel targeted drug delivery system using cationic emulsion-antibody conjugates, J Control Release, 2005, 108, 418–432.

101. Hirsch LR, Gobin AM, Lowery AR, Tam F, Drezek RA, Halas NJ, West JL, Metal nanoshells, Ann Biomed Eng, 2006, 34, 15–22.

102. Corot C, Robert P, Idee JM, Port M, Recent advances in iron oxide nanocrystal technology for medical imaging, Adv Drug Deliv Rev, 2006, 58, 1471–1504.

103. Indu PK, Manjit S, Meenakshi K, Formulation and evaluation of ophthalmic preparations of acetazolamide, Int J Pharm, 2000, 199, 119–127.

104. Mitan R, Gokulgandhi Jolly R, Parikh, Megha B, Dharmesh MM, A pH triggered *in situ* gel forming ophthalmic drug delivery system for tropicamide, Drug Deliv Technol, 2007, 5, 44–49.

105. Sultana Y, Aqil M, Ali A, Zafar S, Evaluation of carbopol-methyl cellulose based sustained-release ocular delivery system for pefloxacin mesylate using rabbit eye model, Pharm Dev Technol, 2006, 11, 313-319.

106. Srividya B, Cardoza RM, Amin PD, Sustained ophthalmic delivery of ofloxacin from a pH triggered *in situ* gelling system, J Control Release, 2001, 73, 205-211.

107. Katarina E, Johan C, Roger, P, Rheological evaluation of poloxamer as an *in situ* gel for ophthalmic use, Eur J Pharm Sci, 1998, 6, 105–112.

108. El-Kamel AH, *In vitro* and *in vivo* evaluation of Pluronic F127-based ocular delivery system for timolol maleate, Int J Pharm, 2002, 241, 47-55.

109. Balasubramaniam J, Kant S, Pandit JK, *In vitro* and *in vivo* evaluation of the Gelrite gellan gum-based ocular delivery system for indomethacin, Acta Pharm, 2003, 53, 251-261.

110. Johan C, Katarina E, Roger P, Katarina, J, Rheological evaluation of gelrite *in situ* gel for opthalmic use, Eur J Pharm Sci, 1998, 6, 113–116.

111. Saettone MF, Salminen L, Ocular inserts for topical delivery, Adv Drug Deliv Rev, 1995, 16, 95- 106.

112. Sultana Y, Zafar S, Ali A, Enhanced ocular bioavailability with sol to gel system of pefloxacin mesylate: *In-vitro* and *in-vivo* studies, J Sci Pharm, 2003, 4, 5-10.

113. Lee YC, Millard JW, Negvesky GJ, Butrus SI, Yalkowsky SH, Formulation and *in vivo* evaluation of ocular insert containing phenylephrine and tropicamide, Int J Pharm, 1999, 182, 121-126.

114. Gurny R, Baeyens V, Kaltsatos V, Boisrame B, Fathi M, Evaluation of soluble bioadhesive ophthalmic drug inserts (BODIR) for prolonged release of gentamicin: Lachrymal pharmacokinetics and ocular tolerance, J Ocul Pharmacol Ther, 1998, 14, 263-272.

115. Hiratani H, Fujiwara A, Tamiya Y, Mizutaniand Y, Alvarez C, Ocular release of timolol from molecularly imprinted soft contact lenses, Biomaterials 2005, 26, 1293-1298.

116. Grzeskowiak E, Technology and biopharmaceutical availability of solid ocular inserts containg sulfadicramide and some promoters, Acta Pol Pharm, 1998, 55, 205-210.

117. Jain RA, The manufacturing techniques of various drug loaded biodegradable poly(lactide-co-glycolide) (PLGA) devices, Biomaterials, 2000, 21, 2475–2490.

118. Brannon-Peppas L, Recent advances on the use of biodegradable microparticles and nanoparticles in controlled drug delivery, Int J Pharm, 1995, 116, 1–9.

119. Uhrich KE, Cannizzaro SM, Polymeric systems for controlled drug release, Chem Rev, 1999, 99, 3181–3198.

120. Mainardes RM and Silva LP, Drug delivery systems: Past, present, and future, Curr Drug Targets, 2004, 5, 449–455.

121. Fonseca C, Simo͂ es S, Paclitaxel-loaded PLGA nanoparticles: preparation, physiochemical characterization and in vitro anti-tumoral activity, J Control Release, 2002, 83, 273–286.

122. Yoo HS, Lee KH, In vitro and in vivo anti-tumor activities of nanoparticles based on doxorubicin-PLGA conjugates, J Control Release, 2000, 68, 419–431.

123. Labhasetwar V, Song CX, Arterial uptake of biodegradable nanoparticles: Effect of surface modifications, J Pharm Sci, 1998, 87, 1229–1234.

124. Lanza GM, Yu X, Targeted antiproliferative drug delivery to vascular smooth muscle cells with a magnetic resonance imaging nanoparticle contrast agent implications for rational therapy of restenosis, Circulation, 2002, 106, 2842–2847.

125. Caves JM and Chaikof EL, The evolving impact of microfabrication and nanotechnology on stent design, J Vasc Surg, 2006, 44, 1363–1368.

126. Seymour LW, Duncan R, Poly(ortho ester) matrices for controlled release of the antitumor agent 5-fluorouracil, J Control Release, 1994, 31, 201–206.

127. Roskos KV, Fritzinger BK, Development of a drug-delivery system for the treatment of periodontal-disease based on bioerodible poly(ortho esters), Biomaterials, 1995, 16, 313–317.

128. Fu J, Li X, Encapsulation of phthalocyanines in biodegradable poly(sebacic anhydride) nanoparticles, Langmuir, 2002, 18, 3843–3847.

129. Calonge M, The treatment of dry eye, Surv, Ophthalmol, 2001, 45, S227–S239.

130. Lin CP, Boehnke M, Influences of methylcellulose on corneal epithelial wound healing, J Ocul Pharmacol Ther, 1999, 15, 59–63.

131. Toda I, Shinozaki N, Tsubota K, Hydroxypropyl methylcellulose for the treatment of severe dry eye associated with Sjo¨ gren's syndrome, Cornea, 1996, 15, 120– 128.

132. Meseguer G, Gurny R, Buri P, Rozier A, Plazonnet B, Gamma scintigraphic study of precorneal drainage and assessment of miotic response in rabbits of various ophthalmic formulations containing pilocarpine, Int J Pharm, 1993, 95, 229– 234.

133. Se´choy O, Tissie G, Se´bastian C, Maurin F, Driot JY, Trinquand C, A new long acting ophthalmic formulation of Carteolol containing alginic acid, Int J Pharm, 2000, 207, 109– 116.

134. Donabedian DH, Martin L, Eng DJ, Compositions comprising cationic polysaccharides and cationic drugs, EP 0 888, 1999, 770 A1.

135. Weyenberg W, Ludwig A, In vitro assessment of the interaction mechanism between mucin and cationic cellulosic derivatives by rheological methods using an experimental design, Pharmazie, 2002, 57, 628– 631.

136. Hui HW and Robinson JR, Ocular drug delivery of progesterone using a bioadhesive polymer, Int J Pharm, 1985, 26, 203–213.

137. Leung SS and Robinson JR, The contribution of anionic polymer structural features to mucoadhesion, J Control Release, 1988, 5, 223–231.

138. Degim Z, Kellaway IW, An investigation of the interfacial interaction between poly(acrylic acid) and glycoprotein, Int J Pharm, 1998, 175, 9 –16.

139. Hartmann V, Keipert S, Physico-chemical, in vitro and in vivo characterisation of polymers for ocular use, Pharmazie, 2000, 55, 440–443.

140. Ceulemans J and Ludwig A, Optimisation of carbomer viscous eye drops: an in vitro experimental design approach using rheological techniques, Eur J Pharm Biopharm, 2002, 54, 41–50.

141. Lehr CM, Lee YH, Lee VHL, Improved ocular penetration of gentamicin by mucoadhesive polymer in the pigmented rabbit, Invest Ophthalmol Visual Sci, 1994, 35, 2809–2814.

142. Saettone MF, Monti D, Torracca MT, Chetoni P, Giannaccini B, Mucoadhesive liquid ophthalmic vehicles: evaluation of macromolecular ionic complexes of pilocarpine, Drug Dev Ind Pharm, 1989, 15, 2475–2489.

143. Oescher M, Keipert S, Polyacrylic acid/polyvinylpyrrolidone biopolymeric systems: I. Rheological and mucoadhesive properties of formulations potentially useful for the treatment of dry-eye-syndrome, Eur J Pharm Biopharm, 1999, 47, 113–118.

144. Marner K, Moller PM, Dillon M, Rask-Pedersen E, Viscous carbomer eye drops in patients with dry eye, Acta Ophthalmol Scand, 1996, 74, 249–252.

145. Setiawan K, Davies N, Tucker I, Patent WO98/47536.

146. Laurent TC, Biochemistry of hyaluronan, Acta Oto-Laryngol. (Stockh.), 1987, 7–24.

147. Wysenbeek YS, Loya N, Ben Sira I, Ophir I, Ben Saul Y, The effect of sodium hyaluronate on the corneal epithelium. An ultrastructural study, Invest Ophthalmol Visual Sci, 1988, 29, 194–199.

148. Ludwig A, Van Ooteghem M, Evaluation of sodium hyaluronate as viscous vehicle for eye drops, J Pharm Belg, 1989, 44, 391–397.

149. Condon PI, McEwen CG, Wright M, Mackintosh G, Prescott RJ, McDonald C, Double blind, randomised, placebo controlled, crossover, multicenter study to determine the efficacy of a 0.1%(w/v) sodium hyaluronate solution (Fermavisc) in the treatment of dry eye syndrome, Br J Ophthalmol, 1999, 83, 1121–1124.

150. Aragona P, Papa V, Micali A, Santocono M, Milazzo G, Long term treatment of sodium-hyaluranate-containing artificial tears reduces

ocular surface damage in patients with dry eye, Br J Ophthalmol, 2002, 86, 181– 184.

151. Gurny R, Ibrahim H, Aebi A, Buri P, Wilson CG, Washington N, Edman P, Camber O, Design and evaluation of controlled release systems for the eye, J Control Release, 1987, 6, 367– 373.

152. Camber O, Edman P, Sodium hyaluronate as an ophthalmic vehicle: some factors governing its effect on the ocular absorption of pilocarpine, Curr Eye Res, 1989, 6, 563– 567.

153. Bucolo C, Spadaro A, Mangiafico S, Pharmacological evaluation of a new timolol/pilocarpine formulation, Ophthalmic Res, 1998, 30, 101– 108.

154. Herrero-Vanrell R, Fernandez-Carballido A, Frutos G, Cadorniga R, Enhancement of the mydriatic response to tropicamide by bioadhesive polymers, J Ocul Pharmacol Ther, 2000, 16, 419– 428.

155. Camber O, Lundgren P, Diffusion of some low molecular weight compounds in sodium hyaluronate, Acta Pharm Suec, 1985, 22, 315– 320.

156. Bucolo C, Mangiafico P, Pharmacological profile of a new topical pilocarpine formulation, J Ocul Pharmacol Ther, 1999, 15, 567– 573.

157. Sandri G, Bonferoni MC, Rossi S, Ferrari F, Ronchi C, Caramella C, Ophthalmic formulations based on ternary interaction systems drug–polymer–polymer, Proceedings 30th, Int Symp Control Rel Bioact Mater (Glasgow), 2003.

158. Saettone MF, Monti D, Torracca MT, Chetoni P, Mucoadhesive ophthalmic vehicles: evaluation of polymeric lowviscosity formulations, J Ocul Pharmacol, 1994, 10, 83–92.

159. Burgalassi S, Panichi P, Chetoni P, Saettone MF, Boldrini E, Development of a simple dry eye model in the albino rabbit and evaluation of some tear substitutes, Ophthalmic Res, 1999, 31, 229– 235.

160. Albasini M and Ludwig A, Evaluation of polysaccharides intended for ophthalmic use in ocular dosage forms, Farmaco, 1995, 50, 633– 642.

161. Verschueren E, Van Santvliet L, Ludwig A, Evaluation of various carrageenans as ophthalmic viscolysers, STP Pharma Sci, 1996, 6, 203–210.

162. Saettone MF, Monti D, Giannaccini B, Salminen L, Huupponen R, Macromolecular ionic complexes of cyclopentolate for topical ocular administration. Preparation and preliminary evaluation in albino rabbits, STP Pharma Sci, 1992, 2, 68–75.

163. Burgalassi S, Raimondi L, Pirisino R, Banchelli G, Boldrini E, Saettone MF, Effect of xyloglucan (tamarind seed polysaccharide) on conjunctival cell adhesion to laminin and on corneal epithelium wound healing, Eur J Ophthalmol, 2000, 10, 71– 76.

164. D'Amico M, Di Filippo C, Lampa E, Boldrini E, Rossi F, Ruggiero A, Filippelli A, Effects of timolol and timolol with tamarind seed polysaccharide on intraocular pressure in rabbits, Pharm Pharmacol Commun, 1999, 5, 361– 364.

165. Ceulemans J, Vinckier I, Ludwig A, The use of xanthan gum in an ophthalmic liquid dosage form: rheological characterization of the interaction with mucin, J Pharm Sci, 2002, 91, 1117– 1127.

166. Meseguer G, Buri P, Plazonnet B, Rozier A, Gurny R, Gamma scintigraphic comparison of eyedrops containing pilocarpine in healthy volunteers, J Ocul Pharmacol Ther, 1996, 12, 481– 488.

167. Bernkop-Schnuerch A, Mucoadhesive polymers, use thereof and method for producing the same, Patent EP, 1998, 1126881.

168. Leitner VM, Walker GF, Bernkop-Schnuerch A, Thiolated polymers: evidence for the formation of disulphide bonds with mucus glycoproteins, Eur J Pharm Biopharm, 2003, 56, 207–214.

169. Marschu¨ tz MK, Bernkop-Schnuerch A, Thiolated polymers: self-crosslinking properties of thiolated 450 kDA poly(acrylic acid) and their influence on mucoadhesion, Eur J Pharm Sci, 2002, 15, 387– 394.

170. Bernkop-Schnuerch A, Kast CE, Guggi D, Permeation enhancing polymers in oral delivery of hydrophilic macromolecules: thiomer/GSH systems, J. Control. Release, 2003, 93, 95–103.

171. Clausen AE, Kast CE, Bernkop-Schnuerch A, The role of glutathione in the permeation enhancing effect of thiolated polymers, Pharm Res, 2002, 19, 602– 608.

172. Hornof MD, Bernkop-Schnuerch A, In vitro evaluation of the permeation enhancing effect of polycarbophil–cysteine conjugates on the cornea of rabbits, J Pharm Sci, 2002, 91, 2588– 2592.

173. Leitner VM, Marschu¨ tz MK, Bernkop-Schnuerch A, Mucoadhesive and cohesive properties of poly(acrylic acid)–cysteine conjugates with regard to their molecular mass, Eur J Pharm, 2003, 18, 89–96.

174. Augustin AJ, Spitznas M, Kaviani N, Meller D, Koch FH, Grus F, Gobbels MJ, Oxidative reactions in the tear film of patients suffering from dry eyes, Graefe Arch Clin Exp Ophthalmol, 1995, 233, 694– 698.

175. Agnihotri SA, Mallikarjuna NN, Recent advances on chitosanbased micro- and nanoparticles in drug delivery, J Control Release, 2004, 100, 5–28.

176. Mitra S, Gaur U, Tumour targeted delivery of encapsulated dextran-doxorubicin conjugate using chitosan nanoparticles as carrier, J Control Release, 2001, 74, 317–323.

177. Tokumitsu H, Ichikawa H, Chitosan-gadopentetic acid complex nanoparticles for gadolinium neutron-capture therapy of cancer: Preparation by novel emulsion-droplet coalescence technique and characterization, Pharm Res, 1999, 16, 1830–1835.

178. Shikata F, Tokumitsu H, In vitro cellular accumulation of gadolinium incorporated into chitosan nanoparticles designed for neutron-capture therapy of cancer, Eur J Pharm Biopharm, 2002, 53, 57–63.

179. Zwiorek K, Kloeckner J, Gelatin nanoparticles as a new and simple gene delivery system, J Pharm Pharmac Sci, 2004, 7, 22–28.

180. Verma AK, Sachin K, Release kinetics from bio-polymeric nanoparticles encapsulating protein synthesis inhibitor-Cycloheximide, for possible therapeutic applications, Curr Pharm Biotechnol, 2005, 6, 121–130.

181. Laidler KJ, Meiser JH, Sanctuary BC, Physical Chemistry, Fourth edition, Houghton Mifflin Company, Boston, 2003.

182. Mathiowitz E, Chickering DE, Definitions, mechanisms and theories of bioadhesion, in: E. Mathiowitz, D.E. Chickering, C.-M. Lehr (Eds.), Bioadhesive Drug Delivery Systems: Fundamentals, Novel Approaches and Development, Marcel Decker, New York, 1999, pp. 1 –10.

183. Peppas NA, Sahlin JJ, Hydrogels as mucoadhesive and bioadhesive materials: a review, Biomaterials, 1996, 17, 1553– 1561.

184. Wu S, Formation of adhesive bond, Polymer Interface and Adhesion, Marcel Dekker Inc, New York, 1982, pp. 359– 447.

185. Hagerstrom H, Edsman K, Interpretation of mucoadhesive properties of polymer gel preparations using a tensile strength method, J Pharm Pharmacol, 2001, 53, 1589– 1599.

186. Mortazavi SA, Smart JD, An in-vitro method for assessing the duration of mucoadhesion, J Control Release, 1994, 31, 207– 212.

187. Jabbari E, Nozari S, Swelling behaviour of acrylic acid hydrogels prepared by gamma irradiation crosslinking of polyacrylic acids in aqueous solution, Eur Polym J, 2000, 36, 2685– 2692.

188. Martin L, Wilson CG, Koosha F, Uchegbu IF, Sustained buccal delivery of the hydrophobic drug denbufylline using physically cross-linked palmitoyl glycol chitosan hydrogels, Eur J Pharm Biopharm, 2003, 55, 35– 45.

189. Inoue T, Chen G, Hoffman AS, A hydrophobically modified bioadhesive polymeric carrier for controlled drug delivery to mucosal surfaces, J Bioact Biocompat Polym, 1998, 13, 50– 64.

190. Helliwell M, The use of bioadhesives in targeted delivery within the gastrointestinal tract, Adv Drug Deliv Rev, 1993, 11, 221– 251.

191. Lehr CM, Bioadhesion technologies for the delivery of peptide and protein drugs to the gastrointestinal tract, Crit Rev Ther Drug Carr Syst 1994, 11, 119–160.

192. Rubinstein A, Tirosh B, Mucus gel thickness and turnover in the gastrointestinal tract: response to cholinergic stimulus and implication for mucoadhesion, Pharmc Res, 1994, 11, 794– 799.

CHAPTER 7

FUTURE PROSPECTIVE

Since conventional drug delivery systems (Oral or IVT) have many limitations in diabetic retinopathy, novel formulation approaches like nanoparticulate system, liposomes, niosomes, ocular inserts, in-situ gelling system described earlier etc may be better alternative for the treatment of diabetic retinopathy. By using these techniques we can produce day to week cost effective patient friendly formulations and also eliminate the complications associated with oral delivery and intravitreal injection. The advantages of these approaches may extend to long term contact along with targeted drug delivery and reduced dosing frequency, easy passage across blood retinal barrier due to nano size, direct targeting of drug to PKC/VEGF receptors, easy administration and patient compliance with low cost treatment. Therefore, novel non-invasive drug delivery may be better approach for the treatment of diabetic retinopathy. We are presently engaged in development of herbal nano formulations, using green pharmacy approach (Preparation of formulation using herbal drugs and biopolymers extracted from plant source without organic solvents) to target PKC/VEGF receptors for the treatment of diabetic retinopathy.

Clinical studies aimed at characterizing the effect of vitamin E in the eye have focused primarily on the potential benefit of vitamin E in age related macular degeneration[1-2], retinitis pigmentosa[3] and retinopathy of prematurity[4].

Vitamin E concentration was found five fold higher than other tissues such as aorta[5] which inhibit the activation of DAG-PKC pathway. So by the use of combination therapy with VEGF or PKC inhibitors we can found good and promising result in low concentration in limited period of time.

References

1. Baynes JW, Thorpe SR, The role of oxidative stress in diabetic complications, Curr Opin Endrocrinol, 1996, 3, 277-284.

2. Gingliano D, Cerellio A, Paolisso G, Diabetes mellitus, hypertension and cardiovascular disease: which role for oxidative stress, Metabolism, 1995, 44, 363-368.

3. Gingliano D, Cerellio A, Paolisso G. Oxidative stress and diabetic vascular complications, Diabetes Care, 1996, 19, 257-265.

4. Asahina T, Kashiwagi A, Yoshihiko N, Impaired activation of glucose oxidation and NADH supply in human endothelial cells exposed to H2O2 in high glucose medium, Diabetes, 1995, 44, 520-526.

5. Chappey O, Dosquet C, Wautier MP, Wautier JL, Advanced glycation end products, oxidant stress and vascular lesions, Eur J Clin Invest, 1997, 27, 97-108.

INDEX

153

* 9 7 8 9 3 8 5 4 3 3 6 4 1 *